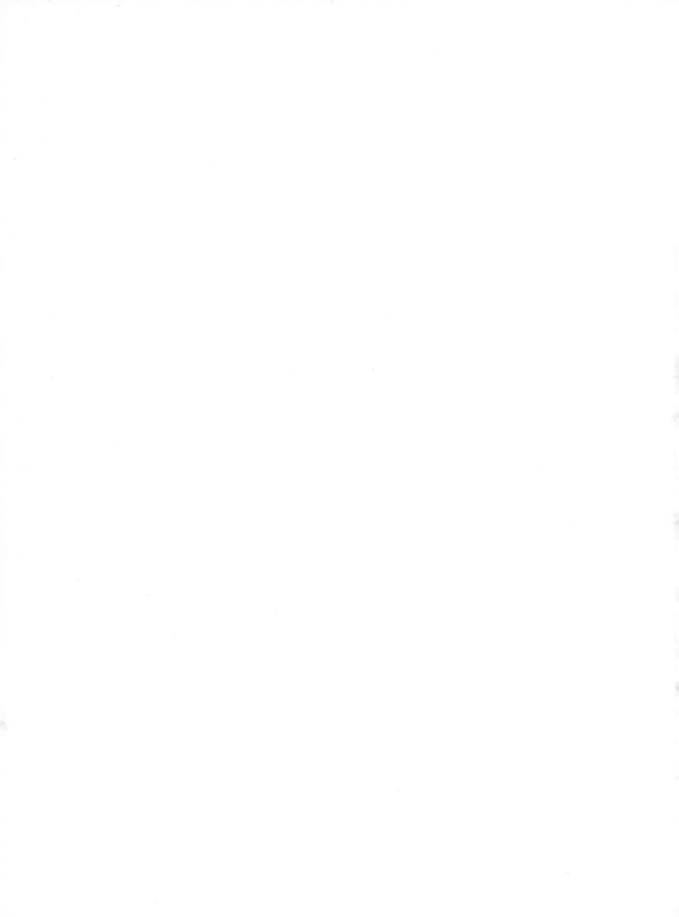

TECHNIQUES IN

THERAPEUTIC ENDOSCOPY

Second Edition

A Slide Atlas of **Techniques in Therapeutic Endoscopy–Second Edition**, based on the material in this book, is also available. Organized into ten topics, each volume of the Slide Atlas corresponds to a chapter in this book.

Presented in durable vinyl binders, each volume in this unique teaching resource consists of text and corresponding 35 mm color slides of each illustration. All the slides are of the highest quality and are clearly labeled, numbered, and indexed for convenient use. The complete collection of ten volumes comes in a long-lasting presentation slip case.

For further information contact:
Gower Medical Publishing
101 Fifth Avenue
New York NY 10003 USA

Gower Medical Publishing
Middlesex House
34-42 Cleveland Street
London WIP 5F B

TECHNIQUES IN
THERAPEUTIC ENDOSCOPY

Second Edition

Joseph E. Geenen, MD
Clinical Professor of Medicine
Medical College of Wisconsin
Milwaukee, Wisconsin
Director, Digestive Diseases Center
St. Luke's Hospital
Racine, Wisconsin

David E. Fleischer, MD
Professor of Medicine
Georgetown University School of Medicine
Division of Gastroenterology
Chief, Endoscopy Unit
Georgetown University Hospital
Washington, DC

Jerome D. Waye, MD
Clinical Professor of Medicine
Mount Sinai School of Medicine
Chief, Endoscopy Unit
Mount Sinai Hospital
Lenox Hill Hospital
New York, New York

Rama P. Venu, MD
Associate Clinical Professor of Medicine
Medical College of Wisconsin
Milwaukee, Wisconsin

Blair S. Lewis, MD
Assistant Clinical Professor of Medicine
Mount Sinai School of Medicine
Assistant Attending
Mount Sinai Hospital
New York, New York

With Original Illustrations by **Susan C. Tilberry**

Gower Medical Publishing
New York ◊ London

Distributed in the USA and Canada by:

JB Lippincott Company
East Washington Square
Philadelphia, PA
USA

Gower Medical Publishing
101 Fifth Avenue
New York, NY 10003
USA

Distributed in the UK and Continental Europe:

Gower Medical Publishing
Middlesex House
34-42 Cleveland Street
London W1P 5FB
UK

Distributed in Australia and
New Zealand by:

Harper Education (Australia) Pty Ltd.
PO Box 226
Artarmon
NSW 2064
Australia

Distributed in Southeast Asia and Hong Kong by:

APAC Publishers Services
30 Jalan Bahasa
Singapore 1129

Distributed in Japan by:

Nankodo Company, Ltd.
42-6 Hongo 3-Chome
Gunkyo-Ku
Tokyo 113
Japan

Distributed in South America by:

Harper Collins Publishers Latin America
701 Brickell Avenue
Suite 1750
Miami, FL 33131
USA

Project Manager/Editor: Toan T. Nguyen
Illustrator: Susan C. Tilberry
Designers: Jeff Brown
Surachara Wirojratana
Nancy Berliner
Editorial Assistants: Alison Marek
Jean Unger
Illustration Director: Laura Duprey Pardi
Art Director: Jill L. Feltham

Gower ISBN 1-56375-018-X

Library of Congress Cataloging-in-Publication Data:

Techniques in therapeutic endoscopy. — 2nd ed./
    Joseph E. Geenen ... [et. al.] ; with original
    illustrations by Susan C. Tilberry.
        p. cm.
        Includes bibliographical references and index.
        ISBN 1–56375–018–X (cased, hardcover) ; $95.00
        1. Gastrointestinal system–Endoscopic surgery.
    I. Geenen, Joseph E. (Joseph Edward), 1935–   .
        [DNLM: 1. Endoscopy, Gastrointestinal.
    2. Gastrointestinal Diseases–surgery. WI 900 T255]
    RD540T43   1992
617.4'3059--dc20
DNLM/DLC
for Library of Congress   91–42602
                                    CIP

British Library Cataloging in Publication Data:

Techniques in therapeutic endoscopy.–2nd ed
I. Geenen, Joseph
616.330757
ISBN 156375018X

Printed in Spain by Printeksa

To our assistants and associates who have given us their support through the years as we were trailblazing. Many accepted therapeutic techniques would not have been developed were it not for your patience, perserverance, and faith—even when we were uncertain.

Table of Contents

Preface to the First Edition

Medical procedures are acquired through a step-by-step process that begins by grasping the concept, watching a preceptor who has mastered the technique, performing the procedure with appropriate supervision, and then proceeding independently, initially with caution and eventually with confidence. While learning, the instructor's ability supports the student. Thereafter every procedure adds to a pool of experience, built on knowledge gained from studying a progressively larger number of cases.

Diagnostic endoscopy requires the physician to combine visual knowledge and perception with some manual dexterity. Therapeutic endoscopy requires special technical abilities as well. Most endoscopists set out to learn a new procedure by observing someone who has mastered the technique, and generally, follow this with preceptor-type training. Once the technique has been learned, it can then be applied in the clinical situation, but questions can still arise as to particular nuances of a standard technique, a special method to use, or how to do a procedure more thoroughly, more rapidly, or better. It would be comforting to have a personal mentor to explain "why," to show "how," to say "that's right," and, once the procedure is learned, to discuss "why not?" or "where next?" Such mentors are not easy to come by and certainly they are seldom around when they are needed the most. Perhaps the next best thing to having such an expert would be a practical "how to" book written by experienced physicians who have not only thought a great deal about the procedures, but also about teaching these procedures. With these concerns in mind, this book was prepared by well-known teachers in the field of therapeutic endoscopy.

This book is intended to be read by the trained endoscopist who is considering the performance of a new procedure or who feels a need for the practical advice of an expert. The endoscopist who has no experience with a particular procedure may, by reading its description here, derive enough information about the technique to decide whether or not to acquire that skill in the time-honored preceptor manner. The clinician who already has some experience will be able to refamiliarize himself with each technique, learn about the latest equipment needed, and glean clues from the experts on how to best approach the procedure, the patient, and how to anticipate and avoid the hazards. Although this book is not meant in any way to substitute for learning acquired in the prescribed preceptor manner, the authors have tried to anticipate as many questions as possible and have addressed all of the important issues.

Although there are a number of books written on endoscopy and on techniques, there is a distinct void in descriptions of the actual practical performance of each technique, and nowhere is there a compilation of the "tricks of the trade" from experts. The need for a practical text is particularly evident when the therapeutic endoscopic procedure is performed occasionally, instead of as a part of the endoscopist's daily routine. By design, this book avoids a discussion of the results obtained and other clinical information that is readily available elsewhere. And, because each of the authors brings his expertise, the chapters are not heavily referenced. The special strength of this book is the unique graphic distillation of the knowledge and experience of each author.

The seven subjects of therapeutic endoscopy covered herein encompass the majority of therapeutic endoscopic procedures performed by the gastrointestinal endoscopist. In creating the book, each author was assigned a procedure according to his area of interest and special skill. Each chapter began as an outline of important information to be covered and, before the complete text was written, illustrations were freely added at each major step of the technique. As the text developed, further illustrations were created to expand each point made in the text. None of the sketches in this book recreates the endoscopic views. All were developed to complement the text or the endophotograph.

Now that the work is finished and each chapter has been reviewed, the impression remains that the text and the copious illustrations represent an amalgam of the visual and cognitive elements required to appreciate any endoscopic procedure. With the marriage of text and pictorial representations, this book on techniques in therapeutic endoscopy provides an up-to-the-minute opus on the many facets of this exciting field.

JDW
JEG
DEF
RPV

Preface to the Second Edition

It has been 4 years since the first edition of this "how to" book was published, allowing trained endoscopists to have their own personal mentor on their bookshelves for easy reference. Step-by-step procedural descriptions were directed to experienced endoscopists who were considering the addition of new procedures to their practices, and/or those who wanted the advice of the experts in making practical decisions. The response was overwhelming.

Since the first edition, the field of diagnostic and therapeutic endoscopy has continued to expand. Areas such as the small bowel and pancreas have been explored for the first time–facilitating accurate diagnosis and treatment. As a result, the topics of enteroscopy and therapeutic pancreatic endoscopy have been addressed in this edition. Once again, descriptions are directed to the seasoned endoscopist who is interested in the applications of these procedures to his practice. These pages, can familiarize one—in a pragmatic way—with the procedure, the type of equipment required, and relevant preliminary "tricks of the trade" from the experts.

In each chapter, the unique experience of the authors shines through to provide the reader with the most up-to-date knowledge on procedural techniques in a clear and readable style. Although there is no substitute for the accepted fellowship method of training, this volume, presented by the experts in a succinct way, will enhance the skill of the experienced endoscopist with the important mechanics needed. It is the perfect complement to the first edition for those who want to keep pace in an ever-expanding field.

Our patients, colleagues, fellows, students, and, especially, our GI assistants have been of immense help in enriching the art and science of therapeutic endoscopy.

JEG
DEF
JDW
RPV
BSL

The Authors

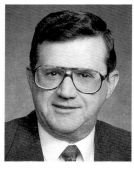

Dr. Joseph E. Geenen is Clinical Professor of Medicine at the Medical College of Wisconsin and serves as a consultant at five hospitals within the Racine area. He is Director and Co-ordinator of the Digestive Disease Center and GI Fellowship Training Program at both St. Luke's Hospital in Racine and Trinity Hospital in Milwaukee. A graduate of Marquette University School of Medicine, he served his Fellowship in Gastro-enterology at the Medical College of Wisconsin.

As a pioneer in endoscopy in the United States, Dr. Geenen has been recognized by many local and international societies. His continued interest in teaching endoscopic techniques has prompted physicians from across the United States and Europe to train under him and observe his procedures.

Dr. Geenen has held numerous positions in many professional societies culminating with his election as President of the American Society for Gastrointestinal Endoscopy in 1982. Presently, he is the Treasurer of the World Organization of Gastroenterology, as well as Governor for the American College of Gastroenterology. At the World Congress of Gastroenterology in 1982, Dr. Geenen received the Bengt Ihre Award in recognition of his expertise in gastroenterology and gastrointestinal endoscopy. In May, 1988, he received the American Society for Gastrointestinal Endoscopy Distinguished Lecturer Award and in May, 1989, received the American Society for Gastrointestinal Endoscopy Rudolf Schindler Award.

Dr. Geenen has been the editor of three books, including the first *Atlas of Endoscopic Retrograde Cholangiopancreatography*, has written more than 90 articles, 20 chapters, and has produced several teaching videotapes.

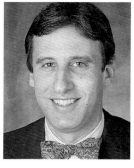

Dr. David E. Fleischer is Professor of Medicine and Chief of Endoscopy in the Division of Gastroenter-ology at Georgetown University in Washington, DC. He received his under-graduate degree from Washington & Lee University and graduated from Vanderbilt School of Medicine.

He is a pioneer in the endoscopic therapy of gas-trointestinal malignancy and his publication on endoscopic laser therapy for esophageal cancer was the first in the field. With Dr. Michael V. Sivak, Jr. and his colleagues at the Cleveland Clinic, Dr. Fleischer participated in the seminal work on videoendoscopy. Other current interests include endoscopic safety and quality assurance, endoscopic ultrasonography, and therapeutic cloggology.

He has written more than 30 book chapters, more than 100 articles, and co-authored a book, *Endoscopic Laser Therapy in Gastrointestinal Diseases.* Two of his teaching videos have won national awards. He has lectured extensively throughout the United States and on six continents.

He has been actively involved in the American Society for Gastrointestinal Endoscopy (ASGE), having directed the National Course at Digestive Disease Week and chaired several committees. He is currently Treasurer of ASGE.

Dr. Fleischer's avocations include juggling, poem writing (low doggerel), sports, and making scrapbooks.

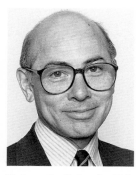

Dr. Jerome D. Waye is Clinical Professor of Medicine at the Mount Sinai School of Medicine (CUNY) and Chief of the Gastrointestinal Endoscopy Unit at Mount Sinai Hospital and Lenox Hill Hospital in New York. Dr. Waye completed his undergraduate studies in Quantitative Biology at the Massachusetts Institute of Technology and graduated with Honors from Boston University School of Medicine.

Renowned as a teacher of endoscopy, Dr. Waye pioneered techniques of colonoscopy without the use of fluoroscopy. He has been deeply involved in the development of new devices and instrumentation in the field of endoscopic technology.

Dr. Waye received the Globus Award for medical writing, a Scientific Achievement Award from the American College of Gastroenterology and, in 1986, the American Society for Gastrointestinal Endoscopy presented him with its highest honor, the Schindler Award. He has received the title of "Master Endoscopist and Teacher" from the New York Society for Gastrointestinal Endoscopy.

He has served as President of the American College of Gastroenterology, the American Society for Gastrointestinal Endoscopy, the New York Society for Gastrointestinal Endoscopy, and the New York Academy of Gastroenterology. He has been Course Director for the National Postgraduate Courses of both the American College of Gastroenterology and the American Society for Gastrointestinal Endoscopy.

In addition, Dr. Waye has written 5 books, over 30 book chapters, and 126 journal articles on endoscopy.

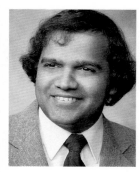

Dr. Rama P. Venu is an Associate Clinical Professor of Medicine at the Medical College of Wisconsin in Milwaukee and is on the active staff at three hospitals in the Racine, Wisconsin area. Since 1980, Dr. Venu has practiced with Dr. Joseph Geenen at Gastroenterology Consultants in Racine. He also has served as Director of the Endoscopy Lab at St. Mary's Medical Center in Racine.

Born in India, Dr. Venu is a 1970 graduate of Kottayam Medical College in Kerala, India, and completed his Fellowship in Gastroenterology at the Medical College of Wisconsin. He is board-certified in internal medicine and gastroenterology.

He is involved in the National Polyp Study with Memorial Sloan-Kettering Cancer Center, funded by the National Institute of Health. Presently, he is involved in collaborative research on the pancreaticobiliary tract and, in particular, on the sphincter of Oddi. He has coauthored 8 chapters on gastroenterology and published numerous articles and abstracts.

In 1985, Dr. Venu was elected a Fellow of the American College of Physicians and the American College of Gastroenterologists.

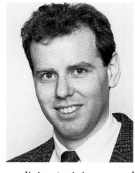

Dr. Blair S. Lewis is an Assistant Clinical Professor of Medicine at the Mount Sinai School of Medicine in New York and holds hospital appointments at the Mount Sinai Medical Center and Beth Israel Hospital North. Dr. Lewis completed his undergraduate studies in Philosophy and Biology at Dartmouth College and graduated from Albert Einstein College of Medicine. His medicine training was obtained at Montefiore Medical Center in New York and he served his Fellowship in Gastroenterology at the Mount Sinai Medical Center.

Dr. Lewis has been involved in the development of enteroscopic techniques and instrumentation. Along with Dr. Waye, he continues their research in the field of Sonde enteroscopy, and together, they have the world's greatest experience. Dr. Lewis has written extensively on the topics of enteroscopy and obscure gastrointestinal bleeding, as well as techniques for the placement of enteral feeding tubes.

Dr. Lewis is a course director for the Mount Sinai Medical School course on the pathophysiology of gastrointestinal diseases. He is on the Board of Directors of the New York Society for Gastrointestinal Endoscopy and the New York Academy of Gastroenterology. Dr. Lewis is presently the Governor representing Manhattan for the American College of Gastroenterology and serves on several committees of the College as well as the American Society for Gastrointestinal Endoscopy (ASGE). He is chairman of the ASGE Scientific Exhibits Committee and is a reviewer for the *American Journal of Gastroenterology, Gastrointestinal Endoscopy* and *Digestive Diseases and Sciences.*

Dr. Lewis was an editor for *Gastroenterology for the House Officer,* and has written more than 35 articles and 10 chapters.

Therapy for Gastrointestinal Bleeding

David Fleischer, MD

1

INTRODUCTION

Endoscopic therapy is the treatment of choice for severe, persistent upper gastrointestinal (GI) bleeding. Although most episodes of GI bleeding are self-limited, medical therapy has been disappointingly ineffective when bleeding was persistent, with a quoted mortality rate of 10%.

Until recently, angiography and surgery were the primary options, but today it is rare for a patient not to have endoscopy as a first line of management. A 1980 National Institutes of Health (NIH) Consensus Development Conference labeled endoscopy "an excellent tool for the differential diagnosis of upper GI bleeding," but suggested that further information was required to evaluate the newer endoscopic therapies. The tone had changed dramatically when in 1989 a subsequent NIH Conference endorsed endoscopic therapy for bleeding peptic ulcers—citing efficacy of therapy and an acceptably low complication rate.

Endoscopic therapy is particularly appealing because it adds the potential of a definitive treatment to the preferred diagnostic method. Most of the causes of upper GI bleeding and some of the causes of lower GI bleeding are readily amenable to endoscopic therapy. The common lesions responsible for GI bleeding are listed in Tables 1.1 and 1.2. This chapter addresses the specific endoscopic techniques used to treat GI bleeding and the preparation that should be undertaken before treatment is delivered.

PREPARATION

Preparation entails localizing the likely site of bleeding to the upper or lower GI tract. Also, determination of the timing of the endoscopy and the specifics of readying the patient for the procedure are necessary.

LOCATION OF HEMORRHAGE

Often, it is obvious if the physician is dealing with upper or lower tract hemorrhage. The medical history of the patient will aid in diagnosis:

- A history of cirrhosis, esophageal varices, duodenal or gastric ulcers, retching before bleeding, or recent aspirin ingestion heightens the likelihood of an upper gastrointestinal (UGI) bleed.
- A history of bleeding after straining at stools or known colitis or diverticular disease increases the odds that it is lower tract hemorrhage.

TABLE 1.1 DIAGNOSIS IN PATIENTS WITH UPPER GI HEMORRHAGE

Peptic ulcers	47%
Duodenal	24%
Gastric	21%
Stomal	2%
Gastric erosions	23%
Varices	10%
Mallory-Weiss tears	7%
Esophagitis	6%
Erosive duodenitis	6%
Tumors	3%
Espohageal ulcers	2%
Angiodysplasia	0.5%
Other lesions	6%

Total more than 100% because some patients had more than one lesion.
(Reproduced from Silverstein FE, Gilbert DA, Tedesco FJ, et al: *Gastrointest Endosc* 1981;27:73.)

TABLE 1.2 DIAGNOSIS IN ELDERLY PATIENTS WITH LOWER GI HEMORRHAGE

Diverticular bleeding	43%
Vascular ectasias	20%
Colonic cancer or polyp	9%
Radiation proctitis	6%
Ischemic colitis	4%
Miscellaneous causes	11%
Source not determined	11%

Total more than 100% because some patients had more than one lesion.
(Reproduced from Boley SJ, DiBase A, Brandt LJ, et al: *Am J Surg* 1979;13:57)

- Hematemesis or blood return from a nasogastric tube means it is an upper GI bleed in virtually all cases.

An otolaryngologic or pulmonary source can lead to hematemsis or cause the nasogastric aspirate to be bloody, but these situations are unusual. If the nasogastric aspirate does not contain blood, it means either that this does not represent an upper GI bleed, the nasogastric tube is curled or improperly placed, or as is the case with some duodenal bleeding, blood does not reflux into the stomach. The finding of bile without blood in the nasogastric aspirate reduces the likelihood that there is duodenal bleeding.

The color of the blood that the patient passes can be helpful in locating the hemorrhage. Bright red blood is more likely to be from a lower GI source, but a very common cause of "lower" GI bleeding is upper GI bleeding, particularly if there is associated orthostasis, so red blood cannot be fully equated with lower tract hemorrhage. Conversely, black stools generally reflect blood loss from a site proximal to the colon, but numerous studies have demonstrated that blood instilled into the cecum can produce black stool, particularly with slow passage. The suspected location of the bleeding will dictate whether a lower tract exam—sigmoidoscopy or colonoscopy—or an upper endoscopy is performed initially. When there is a small but distinct possibility of an upper GI bleed, an upper endoscopy is done first as a quick screening exam.

TIMING OF EXAMINATION

Several factors dictate how soon the examination is performed once the bleeding is realized. If there is active lower GI bleeding, the yield of successful colonscopic diagnosis and treatment is diminished unless the colon is cleansed prior to the procedure. There is usually time to proceed with an oral lavage, such as Golytely® or Colyte® prior to the examination. If there is a high suspicion of rectal source, an unprepped sigmoidoscopy may be useful. If there is persistence of bright red blood per rectum despite lavage and an upper source has been excluded by esophagogastroduodenoscopy, an arteriogram or bleeding scan may be more prudent than a colonoscopy.

With an obvious upper GI bleed several factors influence the immediacy with which the procedure is performed. There are two distinct situations.

- First, is the bleeding ongoing? Red blood per nasogastric tube that does not lavage clear suggests that bleeding is persistent. If this is the case, urgent endoscopy is indicated as soon as, but not before, the patient is medically stable.
- Second, if the bleeding is not thought to be active — lavage clears rapidly, return suggests old blood— numerous factors come into play. The most critical factor is the availability of the endoscopist, the support personnel, and the endoscopic site and equipment. There is a growing trend to avoid middle-of-the-night endoscopy if the patient is not actively bleeding, because the safety of the patient and the success of the procedure is maximized in a less hectic situation.

The patient's physical location is also a factor. With the exception of the rare procedure performed in the operating room for acute bleeding, the endoscopy should be performed either in the intensive care unit or in the endoscopy suite, if the patient is more stable. An emergency endoscopy on a general medical or surgical ward should be avoided because space, monitoring and resuscitation equipment, and appropriate support personnel are generally unavailable. Although policies will differ among hospitals, urgent endoscopy in the emergency room may have similar limitations.

INITIAL ASSESSMENT

The initial management of the bleeding patient should focus on:

- Assessing hemodynamic stability.
- Determining the rate and activity of the bleeding.
- Collecting blood samples.
- Notifying appropriate physicians.
- Moving the patient to the designated site after he is stabilized.

The likelihood of finding the source of bleeding is highest if the procedure is done within 24 hr of the bleed. Other factors that may advance the rapidity with which the test is done are cases where previous bleeding has occurred but no site was found or patients in whom blood replacement is a problem. For patients who are difficult to cross match, who have rare blood types, or who refuse blood transfusions for religious reasons, the surveillance endoscopy should be initiated as quickly as possible. This will allow the most appropriate therapy to be undertaken immediately.

PATIENT PREPARATION

Once the decision for endoscopy is made the physician begins to deal in specific rather than general matters (Table 1.3). The patient's vital signs and mental status will provide information which can predict how well the procedure will be tolerated, what pharmacologic agents should be used, and what monitoring is required during the procedure. The clinical situation will determine what blood studies are required, but one generally requests a pre-procedure hemoglobin or hematocrit, blood typing, and, if warranted, a coagulation profile. Attention is then turned to items that will maximize stability through the procedure:

- Is there good intravenous access and are there respiratory concerns?
- Will sedation compromise breathing?
- Is the possibility of aspiration high enough that preprocedure intubation is warranted or standby capabilities should be aligned?

It is often helpful to notify the surgeon in advance so that he may be on hand in case surgery is needed. He can observe the procedure or, more commonly, can meet the patient prior to an emergency surgical setting. Notification of the patient's family is an appreciated courtesy, particularly in younger or older patients, and at times it is necessary for them to sign the consent form.

Premedication is similar to that used for routine diagnostic procedures. The patient with major GI blood loss may be hypotensive, so the endoscopist must be particularly attentive to the blood pressure lowering effects of commonly used narcotics and sedatives. Antiperistaltic agents such as glucagon may be useful to diminish motility when searching for or treating nonbleeding angiodysplasia. Some clinicians have emphasized that narcotic antagonists may increase perfusion of angiodysplastic lesions and make them more obvious, particularly if the patient was sedated prior to the endoscopy.

At least two support personnel should be present when endoscopic therapy of a patient with GI bleeding is to be done. One will assist the endoscopist while the other monitors the patient. If there is massive upper GI bleeding, particularly of variceal origin, pretreatment intubation is wise. It allows better control of respiration and protects the airway. Intubation is also useful in the combative patient. When health personnel must physically restrain a patient during endoscopy, the procedure carries higher risks. The likelihood of successfully visualizing and/or treating the bleeding source is reduced and the risk of aspiration is increased. The

---

TABLE 1.3 CHECKLIST FOR EMERGENCY ENDOSCOPY FOR GI BLEEDING

1. Are vital signs and mental status stable enough to allow procedure to begin? Is monitoring equipment in working order?
2. Have baseline labs been drawn and checked? Is blood typed?
3. Is there good intravenous access?
4. Is preprocedure intubation required to assist respiration and/or to prevent aspiration?
5. Has surgeon been notified?
6. Have family and referring physician been notified?
7. Has consent for diagnostic and therapeutic procedure been obtained?
8. Are all appropriate endoscopes at hand?
9. Are endoscopic accessories—Water Pik, clot remover—available?
10. Is therapeutic equipment available and checked out?

possibility that the patient might bite himself, the endoscope, or attendant health personnel is an important concern.

SAFETY PRECAUTIONS FOR HEALTH PERSONNEL

Since medical history and examination cannot reliably identify patients infected with hepatitis, human immunodeficiency virus (HIV), or other blood-borne pathogens, blood and body fluid precautions should be used with *all* patients. Health personnel who manage patients with GI bleeding should routinely use appropriate barrier precautions to prevent skin and mucous membrane exposure when contact with blood or blood-contaminated body fluids is anticipated.

Gloves and gown should be worn by all endoscopists for all procedures. If the hands of the physician or nurse are inserted into the patient's mouth, double gloving is recommended. For cases in which the splattering of blood or blood-contaminated body fluids is likely, as in emergency endoscopy for GI bleeding, masks and protective eye wear are essential.

The risk of endoscopy personnel acquiring hepatitis B infection is small. However, with the availability of a safe and effective hepatitis B vaccine, endoscopy personnel should be immunized.

Care must be taken to avoid needle stick injury. Used needles should not be recapped but placed directly into containers. Clearly marked containers for the disposal of all sharp equipment should be available wherever endoscopic procedures are performed.

EQUIPMENT

It is not always possible to anticipate which endoscope will be best for a given situation. In the bleeding patient, the endoscopist must be prepared for massive bleeding as the worst possible case. One large channel—3.5 mm or greater—or a double channel instrument—with a 2.8 mm channel and a second 2.8 or 3.5 mm channel—are generally preferred. The double channel instrument has the advantage of having one channel for suction and a second channel for therapy. Some endoscopists feel both these functions can be carried out by the large single channel instrument. These scopes are sometimes modified to include an additional small wash channel, for either a hand syringe or a water pump or Pik. The range of videoendoscopes available for therapeutic endoscopy is not yet as great as with fiberoptic instruments. It is uncommon to employ videoendoscopy for emergency cases done outside the endoscopy suite, because the equipment is difficult to transport. Videoendoscopy would however provide a valuable record of these acute and difficult cases for review with colleagues.

For laser work, the endoscope often requires a filter to protect the eye and a white tip to minimize damage from reflected beams. Despite the fact that these therapeutic endoscopes have such advantages, smaller diameter endoscopes with smaller channels are often chosen because they are more available. They usually work less well in difficult cases, unless they were specifically selected because the larger scopes cannot pass beyond a stricture or a deformed pylorus. Rarely, in cases of hematobilia or distal duodenal lesions, a duodenoscope is valuable.

Accessory equipment is essential. Just as a thoughtful colonoscopist is always prepared to proceed with a polypectomy if an unexpected lesion is encountered, so should the endoscopist evaluating the patient with GI bleeding be prepared. The physician who undertakes endoscopy for a patient with upper tract hemorrhage should be prepared to treat both variceal and nonvariceal bleeding, particularly if there is active bleeding when the procedure begins. When the endoscopist suspects there is no active bleeding, a surveillance endoscopy will be performed. However, by anticipating the possible need to deliver therapy, treatment can be readily delivered if an appropriate lesion is encountered. Therefore, at the time of endoscopy, the physician should be ready to treat a bleeding site with injection therapy or with one of the thermal devices. Endoscopic sclerosis is the treatment of choice for bleeding varices, although ligation is also being used. Either injection therapy or one of the thermal devices is an acceptable option for nonvariceal bleeding.

Other ancillary equipment should be available. Biopsy forceps may be required for obtaining a sample prior to therapy—although this is usually not done in an acute bleed—but also can be used to remove a small clot which is covering an ulcer just before endoscopic therapy. If treatment is not planned, it is a time-honored view that clots be left in place over ulcer bases. A sphincterotomy basket is helpful to remove a clot and should be kept at hand. A sclerotherapy needle can be used to inject vasoconstrictive agents, such as epinephrine, or vasopressin, around a bleeding site to slow blood flow and improve visualization prior to thermal treatment. Water Piks® can be useful to cleanse the mucosa or to assist with visualization of the bleeding site, if a device without a water stream is chosen.

In order to share what has been seen and done, lecturescopes, cameras, and video equipment are now considered standard items.

SURVEILLANCE ENDOSCOPY

Usually by the time that the actual endoscopy is to be performed, an nasogastric tube has been inserted. It has been standard teaching that lavage with a large bore tube, such as a 34F, be done prior to endoscopy and many experienced endoscopists feel it is necessary. However, more than 50% of bleeding sites will be readily accessible without lavage, and in these situations the addition of lavage lengthens the procedure and fails to provide better visualization. A growing number of therapeutic endoscopists feel lavage should not be done until the upper tract has been assessed by a quick surveillance diagnostic

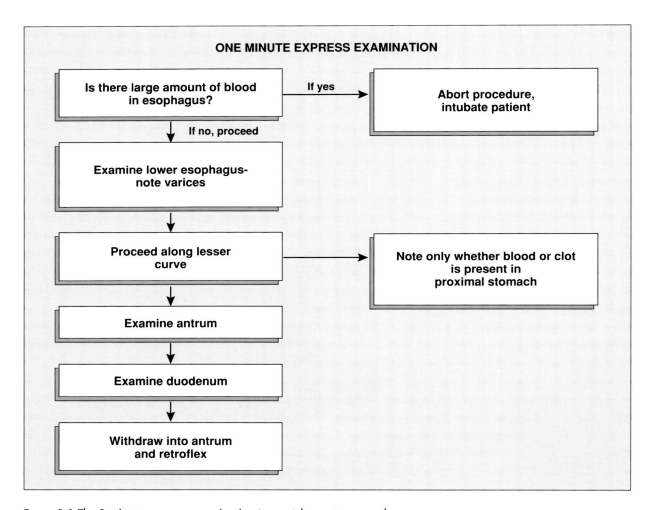

FIGURE 1.1 The **1 minute express examination** is a quick way to assess the upper gastrointestinal tract prior to lavage.

THERAPY FOR GASTROINTESTINAL BLEEDING

exam. An expedient method for such a procedure is the "one-minute express examination" (Fig. 1.1). This quick exam serves as a prologue to the more detailed diagnostic and therapeutic procedure. After the esophagus is intubated, the endoscopist makes rapid assessments:

- Is there fresh blood in the esophagus?
- If the quantity is large, it may be prudent to abort the procedure until the patient is intubated.
- Are varices present? This determination is important because therapy will be different for variceal bleeding.

The scope is then passed into the stomach along the lesser curve and into the antrum. Apart from noting the presence of blood in the stomach or a fundic clot, no attention is paid to the proximal stomach. Antral lesions are generally the easiest to treat. Next, the pylorus is intubated with a quick inspection of the bulb and postbulbar area for signs of intestinal hemorrhage. The scope is then brought back into the stomach where a quick retroflexed view is obtained. This screening can readily be accomplished in one minute and attention can later be directed to areas of suspected bleeding or to the proximal stomach, which is usually the most difficult part of the procedure.

If during the endoscopy a large gelatinous clot is found on the greater curve and no other sites of blood loss are found, attempts to examine that area should be made. Lavage with a large bore tube may be tried. There is little evidence that saline lavage is either safer or more efficacious than tap water, and the latter is less expensive. Unclotted blood is readily suctioned via the endoscopic channel, but even large—3.5 mm or greater—channels for suction do not readily evacuate many large clots. If the clot remains, try repositioning the patient (Fig. 1.2).

In the standard left lateral decubitus position the clotted blood remains on the dependent greater curve. If the patient is moved to the right lateral decubitus position the clot may roll off the greater curve so that it can be examined. When this is done, the risk of aspiration increases. Therefore, this should

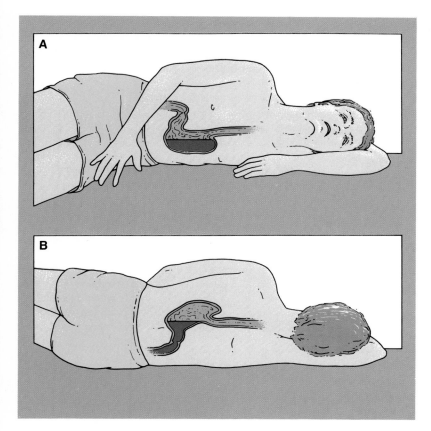

FIGURE 1.2 Gravity can be used to affect the position of the fundic clot. Left lateral decubitus (**A**). Right lateral decubitus (**B**).

only be attempted when the patient's airway is protected.

A gelatinous clot is generally too soft to grab and too hard and solid to suction away. Although no endoscopic accessory is ideal, the large gallstone retrieval baskets occasionally can be useful. Some endoscopists like to insert an overtube so repeated passes don't require reintubation with the endoscope and the airway is protected. Intravenous metoclopramide may deliver the fundic clot distally by increasing gastric emptying, but most clinicians have not found this approach to be helpful. An endoscopic ultrasonic suction apparatus would be marvelous for removing clotted blood, but current technology has not built such a device as yet. If the clot is small—less than 4 cm—it may be helpful to inject a vasoconstricting agent such as epinephrine (1:10,000) around the edges.

If the clot is large and there is no good means of evacuating it, the experienced endoscopist will not spend a great deal of time trying to remove it. Rather, the best approach is to focus on the area not covered by clot and if no other abnormalities are found to repeat the endoscopy the next day. In many instances, the clot will be gone at this time and assessment of the proximal stomach can be accomplished thoroughly in a brief period of time.

ENDOSCOPIC TREATMENT OPTIONS

Several endoscopic methods have been used to control GI hemorrhage. They can be classified as topical, injection, mechanical, and thermal (Table 1.4). Enthusiasm for some methods has swelled as their efficacy and safety continue to be established. The fanfare which initially surrounded some of the others has waned and now they appear destined to become historical footnotes.

TOPICAL THERAPY

Because the agents are applied topically, the risk of systemic side effects or perforation should be negligible, and in contrast to most other forms of endoscopic therapy, the opportunity to treat a diffuse lesion exists. Four main types of topical agents have been utilized—tissue adhesives, clotting factors, collagen, and metallic slurries used as a part of a ferromagnetic tamponade. Yet, despite the appeal of

the concept, none of these modalities has been commonly employed. The major limitations have been the lack of an effective delivery system and the inability of investigators to clearly establish efficacy. The delivery systems for adhesives, clotting factors, and collagen have been cumbersome. There is little evidence that they are effective for spurting arterial bleeding.

Ferromagnetic tamponade is carried out by delivering an iron slurry endoscopically to the bleeding site and then rolling the patient under an electromagnet which is activated to bring the slurry into contact with the bleeding site. The inconvenience of bringing the bleeding patient to the magnet, a piece of equipment not found in most hospitals, has prevented common use of this intriguing approach.

INJECTION THERAPY

Interest in injection sclerosis for variceal bleeding has been great and a natural extension has been to expand the application for nonvariceal lesions. The equipment is inexpensive, the technique is relatively simple and the initial results are encouraging.

Injection therapy has been employed both as a singular form of therapy or in combination with thermal devices. In the latter instances, a vaso-

---

TABLE 1.4 ENDOSCOPIC THERAPY OF GI BLEEDING

Topical therapy
- Tissue adhesives
- Clotting factors
- Collagen
- Ferromagnetic tamponade

Injection therapy
- Variceal bleeding
- Nonvariceal bleeding
  ethanol
  other sclerosants
  epinephrine
  saline
  thrombin

Mechanical therapy
- Snares
- Sutures
- Balloons
- Hemoclips

Thermal therapy
- Electrocoagulation
  monopolar
  electrohydrothermal
  bipolar (multipolar)
- Heater probe
- Laser

constrictive agent, such as epinephrine, is used prior to coagulation. The injected substance will diminish the flow of blood in the artery by a combination of vasoconstriction–created by the pharmacologic activity of the drug–and edema–caused by distention of the injected tissue. Since less blood is present to "carry away the heat," the thermal device will be more efficient.

Several different solutions have been used as single therapies (Table 1.5). Ethanol is usually utilized as a 98% dehydrated preparation. It causes dehydration and fixation of the exposed vascular wall with endothelial cell destruction, wall injury, and thrombosis. Polidocanol is the variceal sclerosant most commonly used in Europe and it is often combined with epinephrine. Other sclerosing agents, such as sodium tetradecylsulfate and ethanolamine oleate, have also been used. Sclerosants cause hemostasis by instigating thrombus formation and also by causing intimal injury. Epinephrine has also been used alone as an injectant and in combination with saline or sclerosants. Epinephrine causes vasoconstriction and enhances platelet aggregation.

Saline has been used as normal saline, 0.9%, or as hypertonic solution—3.6% to 7.2%. Saline is used because it induces edema and vascular thrombosis. It may also prolong the exposure to epinephrine. Thrombin, used with normal saline as a transport medium, enhances thrombus formation by accelerating the conversion of fibrinogen to fibrin.

There is animal data that has clinical relevance. Generally the most effective agents, ethanol and the sclerosant agents, caused the most tissue injury. Because epinephrine works primarily by causing vasoconstriction rather than deep tissue injury, there is concern that rebleeding may occur after initial hemostasis is achieved.

There is also animal data in which injection therapy with ethanol and other sclerosants was used prior to thermal coagulation. Injection therapy, particularly with ethanol, reduces the conduction of thermal energy to the tissue.

MECHANICAL APPROACHES

Mechanical approaches have been employed in selected cases but have not gained wide acceptance.

TABLE 1.5 SOLUTIONS USED FOR INJECTION THERAPY OF NONVARICEAL BLEEDING LESIONS

Solution	Mechanism	Individual Injection Volume (mL)	Total Dose (mL)
Ethanol (98% dehydrated)	Dehydration and fixation; wall injury and thrombosis	0.1–0.2	0.6–1.2
Sclerosing solutions	Thrombosis; Intimal Injury		
Ethanolamine		0.5	2–8
Polidocanol (1%)		1	5
Epinephrine (1:10,000-20,000)	Vasoconstriction		
Alone	Platelet aggregation	0.5–1.0	5–10
with hypertonic saline	Prolongs epinephrine exposure	a,b	1–3
with normal saline			
with sclerosants		c	10–15
with thermal therapy	minimizes heat sink effect	0.5–1	5–10
Thrombin in normal saline	Thrombosis	3	10–15

a=3 mL of a 3.6% saline and epinephrine (1:20,000)
b=1 mL of a 7.2% saline and epinephrine (1:20,000)
c=Inject 5–10 cc of 1:10,000 epinephrine, then 5 mL of 1% polidocanol

---

Clips can be delivered endoscopically to the bleeding site to clamp off the source of hemorrhage. This method requires great technical skill because the clips often dislodge. More recently, a mechanical steel suturing device with a wire helix at its tip has been developed.

On occasion, an electrocautery snare—with or without electrical energy—can be used to grasp a vessel or a polyp stalk that is bleeding. At times endoscopically delivered balloons can be used to tamponade a source of bleeding. In addition, endoscopic suturing has been performed with a sewing machine-like device. These approaches stand more as a testimony to man's ingenuity than as practical solutions at this time, but it is likely that their clinical applications will increase as the technology improves.

Thermal Therapy

The thermal modalities hold the most promise and it is these which have been studied most thoroughly. Monopolar electrocautery was transformed from the operating room BOVIE into an endoscopic modality.

In an attempt to overcome some of the disadvantages of monopolar cautery, bipolar (multipolar), and electrohydrothermal methods of coagulation have arisen. The heater probe was developed in an attempt to harness the combined effects of heat and pressure. Clinical experience using laser photocoagulation has been great and much has been published about its application. To date there has been little interest in the direct endoscopic application of cryotherapy for GI bleeding.

Electrocoagulation results as current flows through tissue near the electrode, heating and desiccating the tissue to form a layer which is broken down and condensed into a necrotic mass. With monopolar electrocoagulation, current flows through the patient to a groundplate. Since this was the only thermal approach widely available for many years, there is much experience using this method, far greater than what appears in the literature. It has been very effective in the hands of skilled endoscopists. There have been, however, some concerns about the method. Depth of injury is great and dosimetry has not been well controlled. Additionally, adherence of

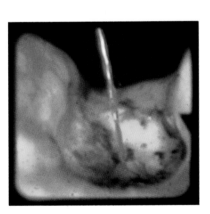

Figure 1.3 Ulcer with single spurting vessel, actively bleeding. (Courtesy of Dr. Marcus Sprintus.)

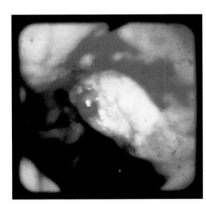

Figure 1.4 Ulcer with non-bleeding visible vessel. This type has a high incidence of rebleeding.

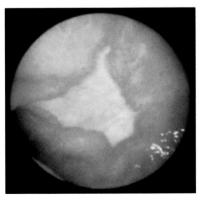

Figure 1.5 Ulcer with a clean base. Incidence of rebleeding is negligible in this type.

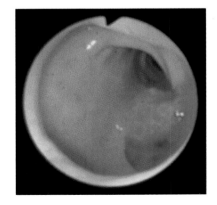

Figure 1.6 Ulcer with fresh, bright red clot on surface. The base of the ulcer is obscured.

the electrode to the coagulated site and of tissue to the probe tip are problems. Electrohydrothermal therapy attempts to eliminate these disadvantages by altering the interface between the electrode and the bleeding site by simultaneous delivery of liquid—water or saline—and current.

Another attempt to improve the efficacy and safety of monopolar electrocoagulation is the development of bipolar (or multipolar) endoscopic probes. In contrast to monopolar electrocoagulation, bipolar electrocoagulation concentrates the current density at the bipolar electrode tip. The tissue contact completes the circuit between two wires only a few mm apart and this limits the depth of penetration, reducing the risk of perforation.

The heater probe was designed to allow the simultaneous application of heat and pressure. It consists of a hollow aluminum cylinder with an inner heat coil and an outer coating of Teflon. The heat coil is anchored in such a way as to insulate it from the external aluminum cylinder. The aluminum's high thermal conductivity provides uniform heat distribution.

The laser provides a light of one wavelength which is coherent and can be sharply focused. To date, only the argon and neodymium:yttrium aluminum garnet (Nd:YAG) lasers have been used for the treatment of GI bleeding endoscopically in humans. A flexible quartz waveguide allows these lasers to be used with the currently available flexible endoscopes. The 0.50 μm wavelength of argon puts it in the visible light spectrum. It is blue-green. The depth of penetration is minimal and it is absorbed by hemoglobin. The 1.06 μm wavelength of Nd:YAG puts it in the invisible part of the light spectrum. It is

not absorbed by hemoglobin and its depth of penetration with combined absorption and scattering is greater. In their initial design, lasers differed from the other thermal devices in one important fashion: the divergent beam could be aimed at the bleeding site from a distance and therefore tissue contact was not required. Laser advocates claimed this made it easier to use the device and that the disadvantages of contact (pulling off clots and the need to be close to the lesion) were avoided. Advocates of the contact thermal methods rebutted that the laser forfeited the critical element of tamponade which increased the efficiency of any thermal technique.

Sapphire endoprobes which attach to the tip of the laser waveguide and concentrate energy at the tip have been designed to expand the versatility of the laser, so that it can be used as either a noncontact or contact device. Refer to Chapter 3 for a fuller description of the thermal modalities.

Ulcers

The majority of bleeding from gastric and duodenal ulcers is self-limited. The appearance of the ulcer at the time of endoscopy has some prognostic significance. An ulcer that has a single spurting vessel (Fig. 1.3) may bleed intermittently. This type, or an ulcer with a nonbleeding "visible vessel" (Fig. 1.4), is more apt to rebleed than an ulcer with a clean base (Fig. 1.5). Rebleeding from the latter occurs rarely. If the ulcer has a clot on the surface (Figs. 1.6, 1.7) the likelihood of further bleeding is intermediate between the visible vessel and the clean based ulcer. If the ulcer has a central red or black spot (Fig. 1.8) the chance of

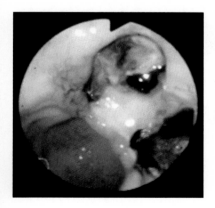

FIGURE 1.7 Ulcer with old, black-colored clot in base. Any ulcer with a clot on its surface has a moderate incidence of rebleeding.

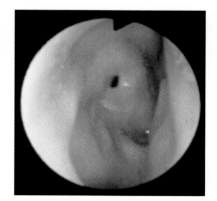

FIGURE 1.8 Ulcer with flat, central black spot. The chances of rebleeding are low but greater than for an ulcer with a clean base.

rebleeding is low but greater than if the base is entirely clean (Table 1.6).

The majority of peptic ulcer bleeding occurs from a single artery just below the ulcer base (Fig. 1.9). Much attention has focused on the concept of the visible vessel. Elegant pathologic studies by Swain, Bown, Storey et al., and Johnston have taught us that what is perceived endoscopically as the visible vessel may represent either a true vessel with a rent in it through which the hemorrhage has occurred, a sentinel clot sitting atop the vessel, or a pseudoaneurysm (Fig. 1.10). Endoscopic distinction is not always possible. In fact, this led the 1989 NIH Consensus Panel to introduce a more generic term, the pigmented protuberance, to describe this finding.

The size of the artery at the base of the ulcer is extremely important, although this is not discernible by endoscopic appearance. The larger the artery, the less likely that endoscopic therapy will control the bleeding and the more likely that surgery will be required. Vessels less than 1 mm in diameter are more apt to be successfully treated than arteries greater than 1 mm. When an ulcer is found on the posterior wall of the duodenal bulb, it is often supplied by a branch of the gastroduodenal artery, and these vessels are often greater than 1 mm. In addition to the fact that they may be too large to be successfully coagulated by any of the current devices, caution should be taken when considering treatment of a nonbleeding visible vessel. All of the thermal devices can induce bleeding and convert a stable situation into an unstable one.

In addition to endoscopic predictions of persistent or recurrent bleeding, there are clinical factors. The greater the blood loss before initial evaluation, the more likely it is that the bleed will continue. Patient related factors are also relevant. Predictors of recurrent bleeding are the association of a coagulopathy and bleeding that occurs in a patient

TABLE 1.6 PROGNOSTIC IMPLICATION OF APPEARANCE OF ULCER AT THE TIME OF ENDOSCOPY

Endoscopic Finding	Risk of Continued Bleed (%)	Incidence (%)
Spurting artery	85	8
Visible vessel nonbleeding	51	26
Overlying clot	41	18
Central red/ black spot	5	12
Clean base	0	36

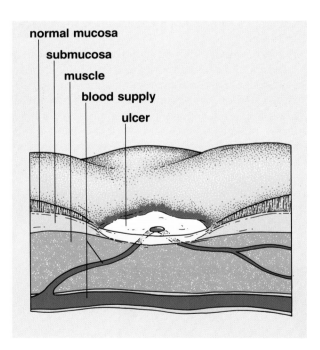

FIGURE 1.9 Peptic ulcer. Note the relationship of feeding vessel to ulcer crater.

already hospitalized. Age and the existence of concurrent illnesses bear a relationship to mortality, but their relationship to continued bleeding or rebleeding is less clear.

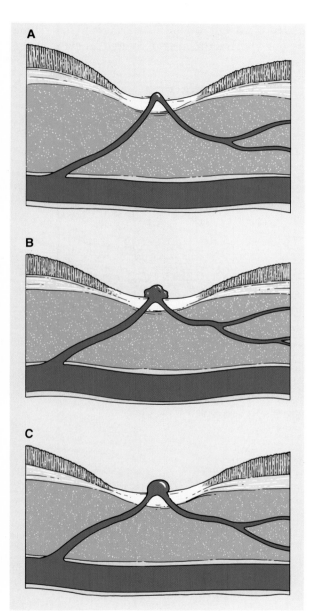

FIGURE 1.10 The visible vessel in an ulcer may represent the actual side of the blood vessel as it pierces the ulcer crater (**A**). A clot on the surface of the vessel is plugging the hole in the ulcer (**B**). Or perhaps there is a pseudoaneurysm of the vessel (**C**).

GENERAL TREATMENT PRINCIPLES

The endoscopic appearance of the ulcer dictates whether or not treatment is delivered. There is general agreement that an actively bleeding lesion should be treated, and that no endoscopic treatment is indicated for an ulcer with a clean base or central spot. There is divided opinion about what to do for an ulcer that has a visible vessel or an overlying clot. Since the likelihood of rebleeding is 40% to 50% for each lesion, some endoscopists feel treatment is appropriate. Others view the same data as support for no intervention. Hopefully advances with endoscopic Doppler, endoscopic ultrasound, videoendoscopy, or other technologies will give predictive information. At the present time, clinical considerations assist with the decision. Treatment should be strongly considered if:

- The initial bleed has been significant enough to cause hemodynamic instability.
- The bleed occurred after hospitalization.
- A single previous endoscopic treatment resulted in initial hemostasis.
- The patient has a coagulation abnormality.

Endoscopic therapy is most likely to be effective when the ulcer base is well visualized with an *en face* view. This is not always possible. With the spurting artery, the precise source may be more readily pinpointed if the bleeding is tamponaded with either the tip of the coagulating probe or a stream of water delivered from either an endoscopic Water Pik or the probes. Therapy can be delivered more precisely if there is no active bleeding.

When a clot is encountered, "gentle washing" is recommended. If it does not come off and endoscopic therapy is deemed inappropriate, the task is complete. If endoscopic therapy is intended for an ulcer covered by a clot, treatment is most effective when the clot is removed. If it cannot be washed away, it will need to be lifted off the ulcer. A double channel therapeutic endoscope facilitates this maneuver. No one endoscopic accessory is ideal. Either a large cup biopsy forceps, a polyp grasper, or a sphincterotomy basket may be tried (Fig. 1.11).

Another approach is to inject a vasoconstrictive agent, such as epinephrine, around the clot prior to treatment. This is designed to temporarily constrict the feeding vessel, so that after the clot is removed the likelihood of heavy bleeding will be reduced and treatment can proceed in a more elective setting. In addition, it may cause enough tissue swelling to unseat the clot (Fig. 1.12).

When a nonbleeding or slowly oozing visible vessel is encountered *en face*, a rimming technique is used with all of the hemostatic modalities (Fig. 1.13). The same principle could be applied with a spurting arterial bleed, but usually visualization in this setting is poor and treatment is delivered as close to the

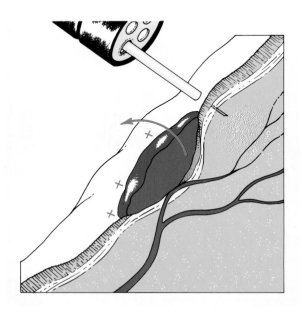

FIGURE 1.12 The injection of epinephrine may cause enough swelling to unseat the clot.

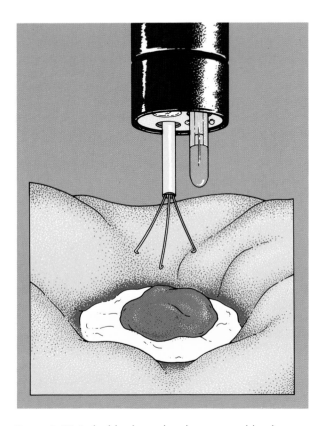

FIGURE 1.11 A double channel endoscope enables the treatment device to be placed in one channel and the device for removing the clot in the other. The clot is first grasped and pulled off. Bleeding may commence as soon as the clot is removed and the endoscopist is thus poised to deliver treatment.

THERAPY FOR GASTROINTESTINAL BLEEDING

origin as possible. There is some controversy as to how close to the visible vessel the rimming should begin:

- One school believes that rimming should begin at the edge of the ulcer base where it is in contact with normal mucosa, arguing that the wider area of treatment provides tissue edema. This edema will temporarily constrict and staunch the feeding vessel and also thicken the ulcer, minimizing the risk of perforation. Treatment can then be directed centrally around the vessel and finally upon it.
- The second school, to which I belong, believes that treatment should be delivered close to, but not on the central vessel—within the ulcer base—arguing that the wide circumference is too far away from

the feeding vessel to be effective and since all thermal devices cause some ulceration of their own, it slows the healing process.

HEATER PROBE/ELECTROCAOGULATION THERAPY

An appealing feature of the heater probe or bipolar electrocoagulation (BICAP) unit is the ability to tamponade the vessel prior to delivering thermal energy (Fig. 1.14). The principle of this coaptive coagulation is that the vessel walls are brought into apposition such that blood flow is interrupted as heat is delivered. This cessation of blood flow prevents the heat sink effect, wherein blood flow carries the heat away and less energy is actually utilized at the intended treatment site. The additional advantage of this touch technique is that one can observe if the mechanical pressure effectively dampens the amount

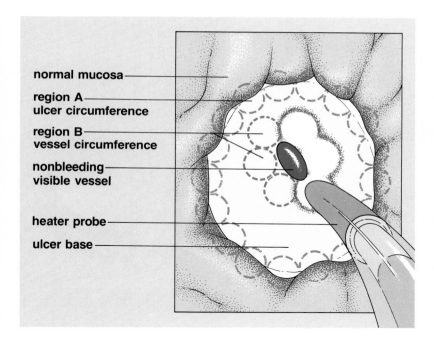

normal mucosa

region A
ulcer circumference

region B
vessel circumference

nonbleeding
visible vessel

heater probe

ulcer base

FIGURE 1.13 With any of the thermal devices a rimming technique is employed when a nonbleeding visible vessel is encountered in an ulcer. Although there is a debate as to whether rimming the ulcer at region A is necessary, it is agreed that rimming should occur around the circumference of the vessel at region B, prior to coagulating the vessel. The edema which is thus formed constricts the feeding vessel, minimizing the chance of induced bleeding. If there is active bleeding, the contact devices are applied directly to the bleeding point in an attempt to achieve tamponade prior to delivery of thermal energy. With the noncontact laser, regions A and B are usually treated simultaneously.

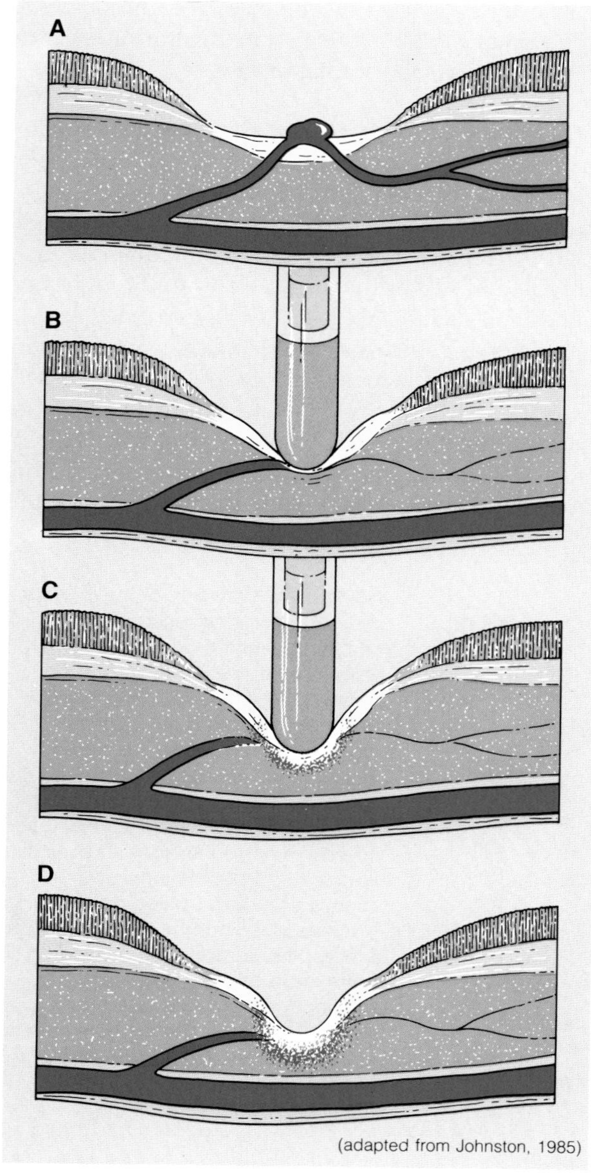

of bleeding, and it suggests the area to which treatment should be directed.

If an actively bleeding ulcer is encountered and treatment is to be delivered with the heater probe or BICAP®, attempt to occlude the site with the probe. When effective tamponade is achieved, coagulation can begin on the vessel. To make sure that the feeding artery has been hit, proceed in a close circle around the initial site. If one encounters a nonbleeding visible vessel, first treat the region around the vessel and then end by directly coagulating the vessel. Although

(adapted from Johnston, 1985)

FIGURE 1.14 Coaptive coagulation. A visible vessel is seen in the ulcer base (A). The contact device is applied to the center of the vessel (B). No thermal energy is delivered. After the device is properly positioned, thermal energy is applied, coagulating the compressed vessel (C). When the probe is removed, a white burn will be seen where the thermal energy was applied (D).

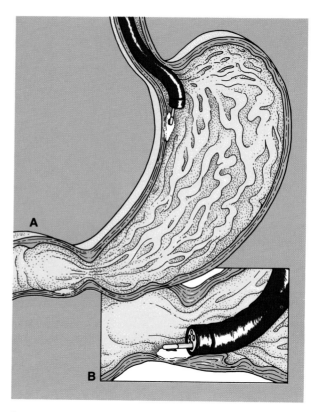

FIGURE 1.15 Coaptive coagulation carried out with the side rather than the tip of the contact thermal device. Side of probe tip used to treat bleeding ulcer high on lesser curve of the fundus (A). With the probe advanced beyond the pylorus, the side of the probe tip is compressed blindly against site of a bleeding ulcer in the bulb just beyond the pylorus (B).

THERAPY FOR GASTROINTESTINAL BLEEDING

many endoscopists recommend circumferential treatment even for nonbleeding vessels, Johnston advocates tamponading the vessel directly.

Often it is not possible to obtain an *en face* view of the bleeding ulcer. This is particularly true for lesions high on the lesser curve or inside the duodenal bulb just beyond the pylorus. In such instances treatment must be delivered without direct visualization (Fig. 1.15). An advantage of the heater probe and BICAP® is that thermal energy can be delivered from the sides of the probes without visualization. Another advantage is that both devices have a co-axial water stream, which is particularly valuable for cleansing the treatment site. Recommended power and pulse duration settings are listed in Table 1.7.

The technique with monopolar electrocoagulation is similar to the above mentioned devices in that the electrode is held in contact with the tissue. Leading proponents of this method suggest that the electrode be positioned 2 to 3 mm away from the vessel and moved circumferentially around it. Depth of injury is greater than with multipolar electrocoagulation. Coaptation is thought to occur in the submucosa and muscular layers, constricting the vessel at that level.

The electrode should not be applied to the vessel directly because the vessel will burst and further bleeding will ensue.

LASER THERAPY

Conventional laser therapy for bleeding differs from the heater probe and electrocoagulation treatment in that it is a noncontact method. The laser waveguide does not come into contact with the tissue. Critics argue that tamponading is logical, necessary to avoid the heat sink effect, and more effective. Proponents state that it is much easier to aim the noncontact device and that it is not always possible to hold the target site in alignment for several seconds as is required with the heater probe. Few comparative data exist.

Initially there was a great deal of controversy as to whether the argon laser or the neodymium:yttrium aluminum garnet (Nd:YAG) laser was better suited for the treatment of GI bleeding. The argon laser, 0.50 μm, with its visible blue-green beam penetrates less deeply, suggesting it would be less likely to cause perforation. It is, however, absorbed by hemoglobin and therefore will not penetrate clots. Although the

TABLE 1.7 RECOMMENDED SETTINGS FOR THERMAL DEVICES

Device	Power	Duration (sec)	Method
Multipolar probe	15–25W	6–14	contact
Monopolar probe	25J	2–3	contact
Heater probe	15–30J	8–10	contact
Nd: YAG			
laser (standard)	70–80W	0.3–0.5	noncontact
Nd: YAG (contact)	10–15W	0.3–0.5	contact

Nd:YAG laser, 1.06 μm, with its invisible beam does penetrate more deeply, perforation—incidence of 1% to 2%—has not been a problem. It has a wider versatility and more than 95% of the lasers used for GI work are Nd:YAG (refer to Chapter 4).

After the ulcer is located and an *en face* view is obtained, the laser fiber is extended just beyond the tip of the endoscope. It should be held 1 to 2 cm from the target (Fig. 1.16). Pulses of high power—70 to 80 W—and short duration—0.3 to 0.5 sec—give the most effective coagulation. If a visible vessel is seen, the beam is aimed circumferentially around it. The endoscopist should wait 1 to 2 minute until edema develops. It will be visible. Then the vessel is treated. A similar tack is taken with an actively bleeding lesion. If a clot is encountered over the ulcer, it is not necessary to remove it. The Nd:YAG laser is not absorbed by hemoglobin and passes through clots.

The laser is less ideally suited for coagulating if the beam has to be aimed tangentially. The rim of the ulcer closest to the laser beam receives large amounts of energy. Therefore, erosive effects and induced bleeding may occur.

One attempt to deal with this problem is the contact probe tip (Fig. 1.17) which can be attached to the standard laser fiber. These sapphire tips serve as lenses which concentrate the energy so that much lower wattages are required. It also converts the laser into a contact device and coaptive coagulation can be carried out. Time will determine if the initial enthusiasm is justified.

Injection Therapy

Injection delivery systems are identical to those used for sclerotherapy of esophageal varices (refer to Chapter 3) Several solutions are available (refer to

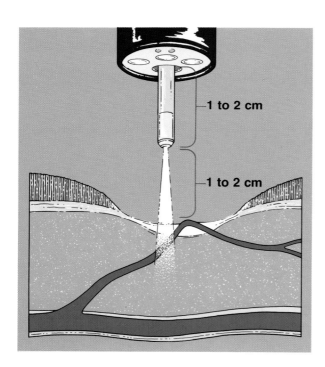

FIGURE 1.16 The laser fiber exits a few cm beyond the tip of the endoscope. The fiber tip is held 1 to 2 cm from the target tissue. The laser beam diverges at an angle of 8 to 10°. The energy density will be greatest at the surface, diminishing toward the serosa.

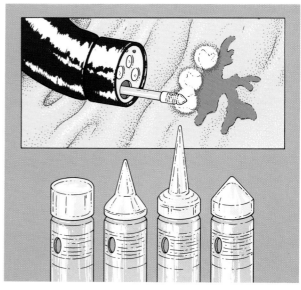

FIGURE 1.17 Sapphire probe tips of varying shapes and sizes can be adapted to the end of the laser waveguide to convert it into a contact thermal device.

Table 1.5). When the bleeding site is obvious–as with a nonbleeding visible vessel–injection is carried out at 3 to 4 sites at a distance of 1 to 2 mm from the vessel (Fig. 1.18). The quantity of solution used is enumerated in the table. When alcohol is injected, some experienced investigators emphasize the necessity of injecting slowly and limiting the volume to avoid extension of the ulcer.

If the bleeding site is not specifically identified, but blood continues to appear at a localized area, there is a role for using an injection of epinephrine, 1:10,000, to "find" the precise site. One cc injections are made in the vicinity of the bleeding site using as little epinephrine as is necessary, but as much as 10 cc may be required (refer to Fig. 1.18). Although the injections are focal, there is some systemic absorption and the heart rate generally increases.

VASCULAR ABNORMALITIES

The nomenclature regarding vascular malformations of the GI tract is confusing. The description of these lesions and their endoscopic therapy in the medical literature is imprecise. Lesions most likely to be encountered by an endoscopist are listed in Table 1.8. Endoscopic distinction between telangiectasias, arteriovenous malformations, and angiodysplasias is seldom possible.

Telangiectasias occur most commonly in the stomach and duodenum, but may be present in the

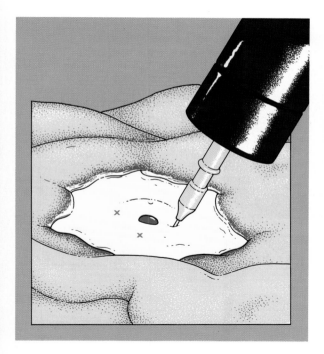

FIGURE 1.18 Injection technique for peptic ulcer bleeding. Injection is carried out with the same needle used for sclerotherapy. Increments of 0.1 to 0.2 mL, 98% ethanol are injected in four quadrants 1 to 2 mm from the vessel. The treated site shows some edema which forms after the injection.

TABLE 1.8 VASCULAR MALFORMATIONS

Telangiectasias
- Hereditary hemorrhagic telangiectasia
- Nonhereditary hemorrhagic telangiectasia

Arteriovenous malformations

Angiodysplasias (vascular ectasias)

Hemangiomas
- Cavernous
- Capillary
- Mixed

Kaposi's sarcoma

colon. They are usually less than 5 mm in size and are often multiple. The lesions consist pathologically of irregular tortuous blood spaces lined by a single layer of endothelium. They are usually capillaries or venules but may be arterioles. No elastic lamina or muscular tissue is present in the vessels. There may be an hereditary predisposition for these lesions (Fig. 1.19).

Arteriovenous malformations consist of dilated thick-walled arteries and nondilated thick-walled veins that communicate. They are most commonly seen in the proximal intestine but can be seen any place in the GI tract. Of all the vascular malformations, the opportunity for angiographic diagnosis is best with these lesions. Early filling veins and dilation of arteries and veins is typical.

Angiodysplasias (vascular ectasias) are usually a few mm in size but may be a cm or larger. They are most commonly seen in the right colon. Microscopically they consist of dilated, distorted, thin-walled vessels lined only by endothelium or a small amount of smooth muscle. Structurally they are ectatic veins, venules, or capillaries. They begin submucosally and, as they become more extensive, show increasing numbers of dilated and deformed vessels advancing through the muscularis mucosa to involve the mucosal surface. Lesions may be single or multiple (Fig. 1.20).

Hemangiomas may be cavernous, capillary, or mixed. They vary in size from a few mm to a few cm. They may be located in either the upper GI tract or the colon. Cavernous hemangiomas are polypoid or

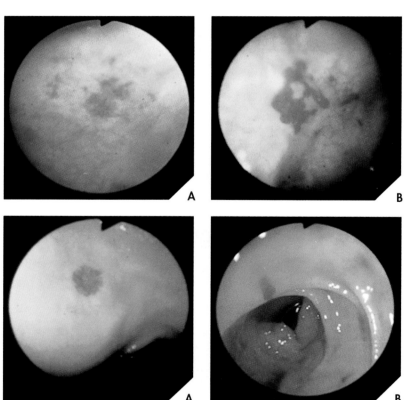

FIGURE 1.19 Multiple, small—1 to 2 mm—telangiectasis in the stomach **(A).** Some have a filiform edge while the lower left one is rounder. A larger 5 mm telangiectasia in foreground with a network of vessels at the 3 o'clock position **(B).**

FIGURE 1.20 Angiodysplasias (vascular ectasias). Discrete 4 mm lesion in cecum **(A).** Multiple vascular ecstasias in ascending colon **(B).**

and histamine-2-antagonists are given postprocedure for upper GI lesions. There is no evidence that they reduce the incidence of rebleeding. Continued endoscopic surveillance is necessary because the vascular malformations tend to recur, particularly in patients with multiple lesions.

ANTRAL VASCULAR ECTASIA

There are several reports in the literature on endoscopic therapy for antral vascular ectasia. The endoscopic appearance can be classic and, when it is, it is hard to imagine a more apt nickname for this

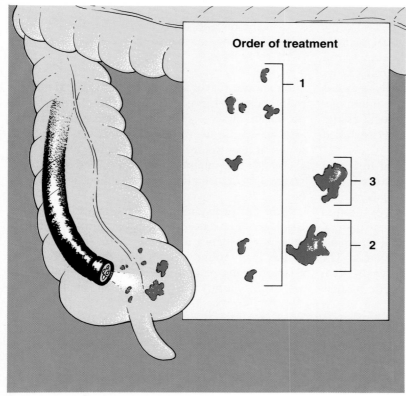

Order of treatment

FIGURE 1.24 Endoscopic treatment of multiple vascular abnormalities in the cecum. Treat all small lesions first because they are less apt to bleed. If there are two large lesions of similar size, treat the most dependent lesion (2), before the other (3). If bleeding is induced by treatment of lesion (2), it will flow dependently and not obscure the field of lesion (3).

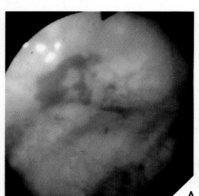
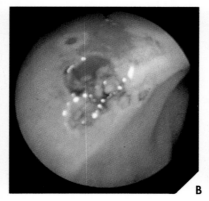
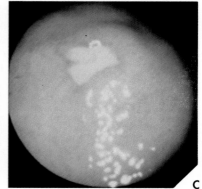

FIGURE 1.25 Endoscopic appearance of angiodysplasia during laser therapy. Untreated angiodysplasia, right colon (A). Immediately after laser treatment (B). Note white thermal burn with some induced bleeding which is self-limited. A small ulcer has formed 2 days postprocedure (C).

condition than watermelon stomach (Fig 1.26). The cause of vascular ectasia is unknown and the supposition that the lesion is caused by trauma in association with pyloric prolapse is conjectural. Histologically one sees vessels of increased caliber, fibromuscular hyperplasia, and fibrin thrombus. The fact that these changes are similar to those seen in association with rectal prolapse support this postulate.

Endoscopic therapy is the treatment of choice and surgery should be employed only if the endoscopic approach is unsuccessful. All of the thermal methods have been used to treat watermelon stomach. If a laser is available it has the advantage of being faster and, since it is a noncontact method, the tissue is less likely to bleed after coagulation. With the multipolar devices and heater probe there is some sticking, which induces bleeding when the probes are pulled off the tissue.

With all the devices, the principles of the treatment are the same. An antispasmodic agent, such as glucagon, should be added to the routine medications to diminish motor activity. If a two-channel endoscope is available it facilitates aiming the thermal devices. Remember that the ectatic vessels are fragile and that treatment-induced bleeding is common. The patient is told before the procedure that more than one endoscopic session may be required, because treatment-induced bleeding may obscure subsequent treatment sites, and that, if too much edema is caused by circumferential therapy at the pyloric, nausea and vomiting are likely to occur after the procedure.

The technical approach is as follows (Fig. 1.27):

- Make a mental note of the pattern of the intended treatment sites prior to delivering therapy.
- Deliver the treatment in quadrants. If possible, treat the dependent (inferior) quadrants first so that bleeding, if induced, is less likely to obscure the other areas.

Remember that if too much edema occurs at the pyloric channel, postprocedure symptoms will be probable. Deliver treatment when antral motor activity is absent—in the gaps between peristaltic waves. It does not matter if one begins at the pylorus and treats proximally or vice versa. The endoscopic image appearance after laser treatment is shown in Figure 1.28.

After the procedure, a H_2-antagonist is used to treat the ulcer caused by thermal injury. Although there is a tendency to believe that a soft diet could be less likely to induce bleeding, this usually is not a factor. If the patient is anemic, iron supplements are utilized until the hematocrit normalizes. If a

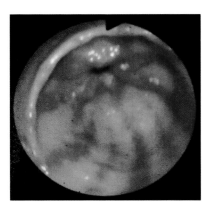

FIGURE 1.26 Endoscopic view of antral vascular ectasia—also known as watermelon stomach.

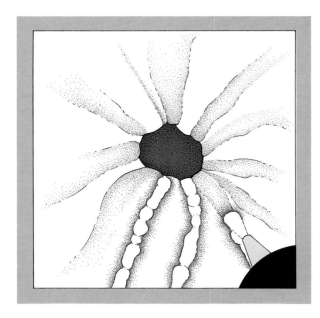

FIGURE 1.27 The technical approach for treating antral vascular ectasia.

second treatment is required, the same principles are followed.

It is important to appreciate that, with long-term follow-up, the watermelon pattern may remain although in a less florid form. It is not necessary to re-treat the patient unless the anemia has recurred or there is symptomatic blood loss.

COMPLICATIONS OF ENDOSCOPIC THERAPY FOR GASTROINTESTINAL BLEEDING

When endoscopic therapy of GI bleeding began to emerge as an alternative to surgery, questions arose concerning safety as well as efficacy. With thermal methods the primary concern was the frequency of perforation. The incidence of perforation is surprisingly low, with rates of 1% to 2% commonly quoted. This is very acceptable considering that the patients are often extremely ill. There have been no notable differences in frequency of perforation with the various thermal modalities.

A more common complication of endoscopic thermal therapy has been induced bleeding. With visible vessels, rates between 5% and 30% have been reported. The incidence with lasers appears slightly higher than with contact devices. Usually the induced bleeding can be controlled with further endoscopic therapy. This can represent a life-threatening complication when large vessels such as the gastroduodenal artery or its branches which supply posterior bulb ulcers are involved. The incidence of induced bleeding is greater than 50% with large vascular malformations although the bleeding is often self-limited or controlled by further therapy.

LOWER GASTROINTESTINAL BLEEDING

The most common causes of lower GI bleeding are hemorrhoids, diverticulosis, polyps and cancer, vascular malformations, and colitis. The treatment of hemorrhoids is not discussed here because it is not undertaken by most GI endoscopists. Endoscopic therapy of diverticular bleeding is not done for many reasons:

- Most often the bleeding is self-limited.
- The diverticulum which bled is difficult to localize, and blood in a diverticulum does not mean blood came from that diverticulum.
- Most important, the bleeding point in a diverticular bleed is, from a practical point, extraluminal and invites perforation.

Polyps rarely cause active, ongoing bleeding and if they do, the principles of polypectomy discussed in Chapter 10 apply. The problem of bleeding cancers is addressed in Chapter 4. The treatment of vascular malformations has been discussed above. Bleeding from chronic colitis—ulcerative colitis or radiation injury—is usually not managed endoscopically. However, in some patients with recurrent hematochezia, coagulation of prominent telangiectatic points is very useful.

There are significant differences between the management of upper and lower GI bleeding by endoscopic therapy. The colon is thinner and thus the risk of perforation is greater. The risk can be minimized by avoiding overdistention. Access to the lesion can be more difficult because positioning the colonoscope may be problematic. Exquisite attention

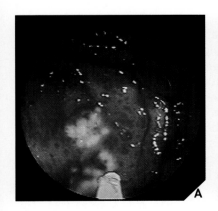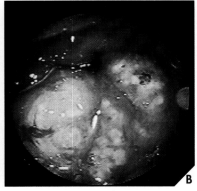

FIGURE 1.28 Endoscopic views of watermelon stomach after laser treatment. Laser fiber is seen at the 6 o'clock position. White coagulation changes are noted (**A**). A close-up image shows the effects of treatment close to the pylorus. Note that the burns are not delivered in 360° to avoid circumferential edema which may cause gastric obstruction (**B**).

to preparation is mandatory. In general bowel cleansing carried out over 3 to 5 hrs with oral ingestion of balanced electrolyte solutions is the preparation of choice. All of the hemostatic modalities that have been used in the upper GI tract have been used in the lower digestive tract with success.

A final note relates to the sequencing of endoscopic evaluation and therapy in the patient who presents with red or maroon blood per rectum and a lower GI bleeding source is suspected. After the patient is stabilized, a review of clinical parameters will set the algorithm:

- If the patient has had a previous GI bleed from a lower source, such as diverticulosis, that will be relevant.
- Is the blood bright, associated with defecation, or other symptoms typical of hemorrhoidal disease?
- Is there associated diarrhea or a history of inflammatory bowel disease to suggest an inflammatory process in the colon?

These clues point to a colorectal source. In elderly patients, both ischemic bowel disease and vascular malformations are common. The association between aortic stenosis and arteriovenous malformations (AVMs) is less certain than was previously suspected.

It must be appreciated that an upper GI bleed may present with hematochezia. Therefore, an upper site is a more prominent consideration when there is a history of ulcer disease, epigastric pain, and bleeding in the setting of orthostasis.

If the patient presents with hematochezia, is clinically stable and the bleeding appears to have stopped:

- Obtain appropriate lab reports—hematocrit or hemoglobin, coagulation studies, type/screen.
- Follow serial vital signs and hematocrits.
- Plan to perform a colonoscopy the next day after a bowel prep with an oral purgative (Colyte® or Golytely®). Although in a classic setting of a "typical hemorrhoidal bleed" one can argue that only a flexible sigmoidoscopy is required, it is my own practice to evaluate the full colon if the bleeding has been significant enough to require hospitalization.

For the patient who presents with red or maroon blood per rectum and who is not stable, the approach is more complex. It is best to coordinate the

management with the surgeon and the angiographer as soon as the patient arrives in the emergency room, the intensive care unit or the general medical-surgical floor. Measures aimed at hemodynamic stability are performed and blood work sent. If the physical examination does not reveal limitations to diagnostic evaluation (acute abdomen), a sigmoidoscopic exam is performed first. The test is designed to answer the questions:

- Is active bleeding seen?
- What is the color of the blood?
- Does the patient have hemorrhoids and what is their appearance? (Often an anoscopic exam will be complementary.)
- Does the mucosa appear healthy or are there signs of colitis?

More often than not, the exam is limited by blood and/or stool and all one can establish with certainty is that there is "blood coming from above the area of the examined segment." If that is the case, then attention is turned to the upper GI tract. A nasogastric tube is inserted. If there is evidence of upper tract blood, endoscopy is mandatory. If there is no blood in the nasogastric aspirate, the next step is more debatable. I tend to err on the side of performing upper endoscopy since it will reveal the cause of bleeding in about 10% of such patients and because the management will be entirely different than if there is a colonic or intestinal source. The decision is based on the answers to the initial set of clinical questions that were asked. I feel that it is clearly mandated if the patient has a history of ulcer disease or if he is hemodynamically unstable.

If the upper endoscopy is nonrevealing, or a decision is made to forego the endoscopy, the next step is based on the presumed status of the patient's bleeding. If there are indications that it has abated and the patient is stable, a semi-elective colonoscopy should be scheduled. If the bleeding is ongoing, my preference is to proceed with angiography. It is my belief that tagged red blood cell scans are more often negative or misleading than helpful. This is being borne-out by growing literature. I believe their popularity can be ascribed to enthusiastic initial reports, the fact that they are "noninvasive" and perhaps more important, they keep the endoscopist and angiographer from being awakened in the middle of the night. It has become conventional wisdom in most hospitals to have the RBC-scan precede the angiogram. I object to this policy because they are seldom helpful, delay the more productive angiography, and often place an acutely ill, unstable patient in an isolated nuclear medicine area without appropriate physician or nursing support.

In most hospitals, RBC-scans will be done nonetheless and may guide evaluation and therapy. Assuming it is not helpful and the patient continues to bleed, arteriography of the superior and inferior mesenteric vessels and celiac vessels should be carried out. If a bleeding site is found, therapy with embolization or a vasoconstrictive drug can be used. If no source is found, I believe it is reasonable to leave the catheter in place for 48 hr since the bleeding may be intermittent.

At this point, in almost all cases a bleeding site has been found or the patient has stopped bleeding. If the bleeding has stopped, the work-up can continue in a more elective fashion. If an adequate colonoscopy and upper endoscopy have been performed, I proceed with a small bowel series. Although the yield is low, it is part of the standard work-up. In the appropriate setting a Meckel's scan can be considered, although I have personally never made that diagnosis.

Assuming all the above tests are nonrevealing, the evaluation usually stops if this has been the first bleeding episode. The patient is then followed clinically. If similar bleeding recurs and no source is found with the previously described algorithm, endoscopy of the small bowel should be accomplished. This is addressed in Chapter 6.

REFERENCES

Boley SJ, DiBase A, Brandt LJ, and Sammartano RJ: Lower intestinal bleeding in the elderly. *Am J Surg* 1979;13:57.

Ertan A, Hollander A: Vascular malformations of the gastrointestinal tract. *Surv of Digestive Dis* 1985;3:42.

Fleischer DE: Endoscopic control of upper gastrointestinal bleeding. *J Clin Gastroenterol* 1990;12(suppl):41.

Johnston J: Endoscopic thermal treatment of upper gastrointestinal bleeding. *Endoscopy Rev* 1985;3:12.

Proceedings of the Consensus Conference on Therapeutic Endoscopy in Bleeding Ulcers. *Gastrointest Endosc* 1990;36(suppl)1.

Silverstein FE, Gilbert DA, Tedesco FJ et al: The national ASGE survey on upper gastrointestinal bleeding. *Gastrointest Endosc* 1981;27:73.

Swain CP, Storey DW, Bown SG et al: Nature of the bleeding vessel in recurrently bleeding gastric ulcers. *Gastroenterology* 1986;90:595.

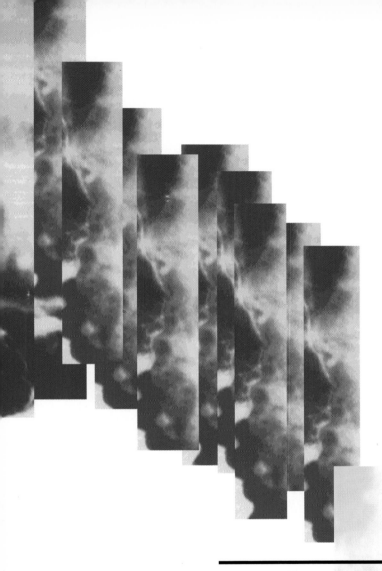

Esophageal Dilation

David Fleischer, MD

2

INTRODUCTION

The association between a patient who presents to an emergency room with chest pain caused by a meat impaction in an obstructed esophagus and a small town in Algeria is admittedly obtuse. In the 16th century, the people of Boujiyah, a mercantile center in Northern Africa, produced tapered wax candles (Fig. 2.1). These candles were some of the first recorded "instruments" utilized medically to dilate strictures, and hence the name bougienage. The first cases of esophageal dilation were not performed with cylindrical tapered polyvinyl devices, but rather candles, whalebones, and other natural products. Although these original dilators are no longer used today, the procedure, bougienage of the esophagus, is still performed in a similar fashion. And though the description of the procedure to the average lay person still seems a bit barbaric, a wide variety of patients with structural and functional obstruction have obtained great relief from this technique.

DISEASES REQUIRING ESOPHAGEAL DILATION

It is helpful to classify the diseases which may require esophageal dilation into 3 categories:

- Benign strictures.
- Malignant strictures.
- Neuromuscular disorders.

A long catalogue of all the benign esophageal diseases which can cause dysphagia can be found in any textbook of gastrointestinal diseases. In some conditions such as candida esophagitis, medical therapy with an antifungal agent is the first step and

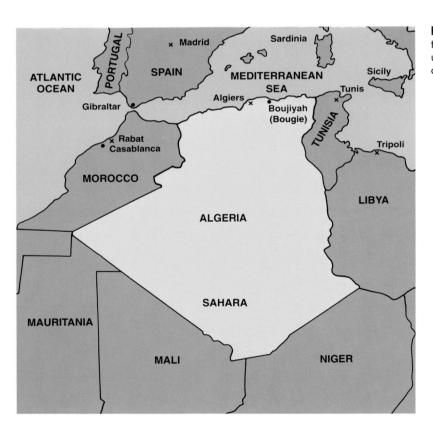

FIGURE 2.1 Map of Algeria showing town of Boujiyah, where wax candles used as dilators were made centuries ago.

esophageal dilation has little role. There are certain benign esophageal diseases for which bougienage is valuable. These conditions are listed in Table 2.1.

BENIGN CONDITIONS

PEPTIC STRICTURES

Most commonly stenoses related to the reflux of gastric and intestinal contents are attributed to acid injury. In certain situations, such as in patients who have had total or partial gastric resections, alkaline injury may contribute to stricturing. Recent studies have shed light on the pathophysiology of acid injury to the esophagus and newer pharmacologic treatment regimens have been extremely valuable. It is now appreciated that a high percentage of patients with Barrett's esophagus with and without strictures produce increased amounts of gastric acid. Recent information also suggests that a subgroup of patients with peptic strictures who do not have Barrett's are hypersecretors. The amount of acid suppression required for effective management of esophagitis is more than necessary for the treatment of ulcer disease.

The practical implications of this data are that it may be useful to measure acid secretion in patients with peptic esophageal strictures to determine if greater than normal doses of acid suppressing medications are necessary. There is little question that acid-suppression with either omeprazole or H_2-antagonists is a critical part of managing acid-peptic strictures. If acid secretion is shut down, the recurrence of strictures may be prevented or the duration between dilations can be prolonged. In some cases, the strictures resolve without dilation when acid secretion is eliminated.

Acid reflux-related strictures always occur at the squamo-columnar junction regardless of its location. Endoscopic views of peptic strictures are seen in Figure 2.2. The stricture is seen 30 cm from the incisors in association with Barrett's esophagus (Fig. 2.2A). Narrowing is seen just above the level of the diaphragm (Fig 2.2B).

CORROSIVE INJURIES

The most common corrosive injury of the esophagus is caused by the ingestion of strong alkali agents such as those found in liquid cleaning agents. The majority of cases occur in young children, but they may be seen in adults who mistakenly ingest material stored in a beverage container or who attempt suicide. The absence of burns in the mouth and pharynx after a suspected ingestion usually indicates that there are no burns in the esophagus. When the mouth is damaged, the extent of injury in the esophagus cannot be predicted without evaluation.

IATROGENIC

Radiation/Chemotherapy. Radiation to the thorax for either esophageal cancer or other chest pathology may result in esophageal injury, although the

---

Table 2.1 Esophageal Diseases Requiring Dilation

Benign conditions
- Peptic strictures
- Corrosive injuries
- Iatrogenic
    Radiation/chemotherapy
    Post procedure
    Pill-induced
- Webs, rings

Malignant conditions
Neuromuscular disorders

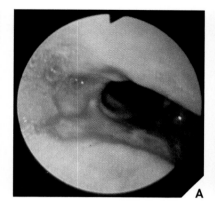

FIGURE 2.2 Endoscopic view of benign esophageal stricture in association with Barrett's esophagus (A).

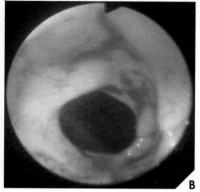

Endoscopic view of peptic stricture at 38 cm from incisors (B).

occurrence is less common now that the portals of entry have been better defined. Radiation injury may produce both structural and motor abnormalities. The likelihood of damage is greater with increased doses of radiation. Problems are seldom seen with less than 3,000 rad (30 GY). Esophagitis with eventual stricturing becomes more common after 5,000 to 6,000 rads (50 to 60 GY). Strictures usually form months after injury but may occur as early as a few weeks after epithelial injury. It is postulated that prostaglandin metabolites are involved in radiation damage. Inhibitors of cyclo-oxygenase enzymes such as indomethacin have been used to protect the esophagus from damage with some modest benefit. Dysphagia in patients receiving radiation may also be caused by motility disorders associated with smooth muscle damage and reduced lubrication if the salivary and parotid glands are injured when the head and neck are in the treatment field.

Esophageal damage is likely to be more serious when certain chemotherapeutic agents are given in combination with mediastinal radiation. Chemotherapy potentiates the effect of radiation so injury may occur with doses less than 3,000 rads. Esophageal injury and stricture formation have been associated with adriamycin, bleomycin, fluorouracil, methotrexate, cisplatin, and etoposide.

POSTTHERAPY

Variceal sclerotherapy. Stricture formation following sclerotherapy for esophageal varices may occur in 20% to 50% of patients. Strictures may develop as early as 2 weeks after injection. They have been associated with all agents. Submucosal fibrosis is probably more important than impaired acid clearance as a mechanism. Neither acid suppression, anti-reflux measures, nor sucralfate slurries predictably impede stricture formation.

Tumor probe therapy. Since its development in 1985, the BICAP® tumor probe has been used to treat esophageal cancer (refer to Chapter 4). Initially it was felt that perforation or hemorrhage would be the most frequent major complication. With increased use of this device, it has been appreciated that stricture formation is the most common adverse reaction (Fig. 2.3). When normal tissue is burned. There is intense collagen deposition and the stricture may be extremely tight.

Pill-induced. Esophageal injury caused by pill ingestion may occur in an area above a narrowed segment of the esophagus but it can also be seen when there is no pre-existing disease. The injury most commonly occurs above the aortic arch and can be caused by taking the pill with too little water or while lying down. Commonly, ulceration forms and odynophagia is the predominant symptom. Stricture formation may also be seen. The most common medications associated with this problem are tetracycline, potassium, and quinidine.

WEBS, RINGS

Esophageal webs are membrane-like structures covered by squamous epithelium. They are usually in the cervical esophagus. They may be single or multiple. They may be missed at endoscopy because they are not obvious or because the endoscope

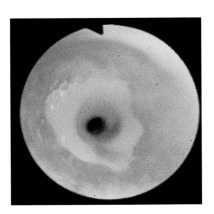

FIGURE 2.3 Endoscopic view of tight circumferential stricture caused by burn to normal esophageal tissue by BICAP tumor probe at proximal margin of neoplasm.

ESOPHAGEAL DILATION

ruptures the web in the blind passage between the cricopharyngeus and the upper-mid esophagus.

The most common ring is the lower esophageal "B" (Schatzki) ring (Fig. 2.4). It forms at the squamo-columnar junction and is seen in association with hiatal hernia. It is a frequent cause of intermittent dysphagia.

MALIGNANT CONDITIONS

Squamous cell carcinoma is the most common malignancy of the esophagus, but any esophageal malignancy can lead to dysphagia. Although esophageal malignancies in two different patients may appear the same histologically, they may respond differently to dilation. Rubbery elastic tumors can be stretched, but the dilation seldom translates to clinical benefit. There is also little benefit gained from dilating extra-esophageal neoplasms, such as pulmonary, that narrow the lumen and cause dysphagia.

NEUROMUSCULAR DISORDERS

Achalasia is the main neuromuscular disorder for which dilation is utilized, although numerous other conditions such as myasthenia gravis, polymyositis, and muscular dystrophy may cause dysphagia. There are anecdotal reports of dilation improving swallowing in patients with diffuse esophageal spasm

and hyperdynamic ("nutcracker") esophagus. Bougienage may also be useful in scleroderma, but only when a peptic stricture forms because of the low pressure in the distal esophageal sphincter occurring in combination with poor acid clearance. A condition affecting the upper esophageal sphincter termed cricopharyngeal achalasia may cause dysphagia, but dilation is not of value.

Therefore, classic achalasia–a motor condition defined by failure of the lower esophageal sphincter (LES) to completely relax, increased LES pressure, and absence of esophageal peristalsis–is the only neuromuscular condition for which dilation is commonly employed. It is usually idiopathic but the manometric findings described above have been seen in association with systemic disorders such as amyloidosis and a wide variety of malignancies. There have been some reports of successful medical therapy and esophagomyotomy has been used frequently, but esophageal dilation is the most common treatment.

EVALUATION OF DYSPHAGIA

The cause of dysphagia is often apparent from the patient's history. A male alcoholic smoker who describes weight loss in association with progressive dysphagia—worse for solids than liquids—is likely to have esophageal cancer. A young patient with symptoms of esophageal reflux with no risk factors for cancer is more likely to have a peptic stricture. The

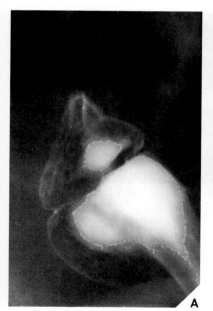

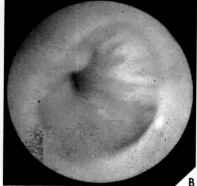

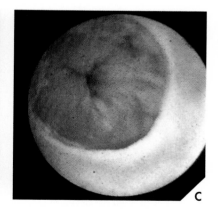

FIGURE 2.4. Esophagram **(A)** and endoscopic images **(B** and **C)** from a patient demonstrating typical appearance of Schatzki's ring. (Courtesy of Dr. Stanley Benjamin)

history will often define the order and number of diagnostic studies that are performed to solidify the diagnosis, but 3 tests are generally employed:

- Contrast radiograph.
- Upper endoscopy.
- Motility studies.

In some instances, especially when cancer is being considered, an imaging study such as a CT scan of the chest and upper abdomen or an endoscopic ultrasound will be employed. This latter study may also be useful when the three main tests do not reveal an etiology and an extra esophageal disease is strongly considered.

The contrast radiograph is generally performed as an esophagram or upper GI series with barium as a liquid. For complicated cases, particularly when a motility disorder or a disease of the hypopharynx or cervical esophagus is being considered, the use of a video tape as opposed to spot films will be helpful so that the dynamics can be reviewed. It is also well appreciated that liquid barium may not reproduce the clinical situation. Therefore, the use of standardized barium tablets may be extremely valuable. Most commonly a 13 mm pill is utilized because 13 mm is generally quoted as being the diameter below which dysphagia will occur.

The upper endoscopy combines direct observation with the additional benefit of acquiring tissue samples. With an endoscopic biopsy a final diagnosis can often be guaranteed. Since most endoscopes are less than 13 mm in diameter, no resistance may be encountered and therefore a subtle narrowing could

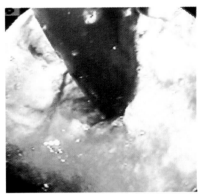

FIGURE 2.6 Endoscopic view of cardia of the stomach shown with instrument retroflexed. An adenocarcinoma in proximal stomach is cause of dysphagia.

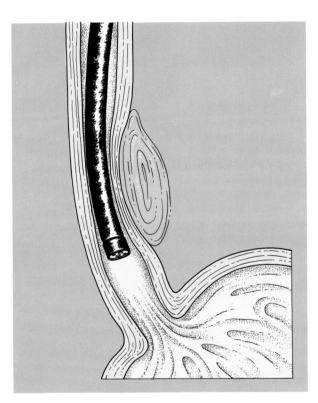

FIGURE 2.5 Slim diameter endoscope advancing easily through esophagus. Luminal narrowing due to pulmonary neoplasm is not appreciated because mucosa is normal and diminuition of esophageal diameter, though small enough to cause dysphagia, does not impair passage of instrument.

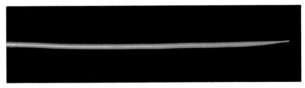

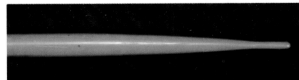

FIGURE 2.7 Maloney dilators are made of rubber and filled with mercury. The tip is tapered.

be missed (Fig. 2.5). In addition, the scope is being advanced with some control and force distally and, therefore, it may pass when food would not. Although most causes of dysphagia reside in the esophagus, it is important to perform a retroflex view after the endoscope has entered the stomach to make sure the cardia is viewed so as to exclude a cause of dysphagia in the proximal stomach (Fig. 2.6).

If the barium study and upper endoscopy do not reveal a cause for dysphagia, then a motility study is usually indicated. Motor abnormalities are more likely to explain the cause of dysphagia when there is more difficulty with liquids than solids, when symptoms are intermittent and not progressive, and when there is intermittent chest pain. Standard motility testing is performed as an individual study and the use of provocative testing may increase the yield. When the symptoms are more intermittent, 24-hr testing may be of value.

It is seldom that the three above tests will not yield an explanation of dysphagia, but if they do not, consideration should be given to an imaging study such as a CT scan or endoscopic ultrasound. The focus in searching for a cause of dysphagia with these tests is to find extra esophageal disease. If the diagnosis of esophageal cancer has been made, these tests would be useful for staging.

INSTRUMENTS

DILATORS

Although wax and whalebone were used many years ago and metal and woven silk were employed in the last decade, at this time dilators are of 3 basic types:

- Rubber mercury filled dilators.
- Tapered polyvinyl dilators.
- Balloon dilators.

In some situations, one type is clearly preferable to the others. For achalasia, balloon dilators are used almost exclusively and the tapered polyvinyl bougies are most effective for malignant strictures. However in many situations, all types of dilators would be satisfactory and it is only a matter of personal preference or local convention that dictates what is chosen.

Mercury-filled bougies. The concept of the weighted bougie is 200 years old. Initially lead was used. Hurst described the blunt tipped rubber mercury filled dilator in 1915. A variation on this theme was the tapered version described by Maloney which is commonly employed today (Fig. 2.7). It is particularly satisfactory for reflux related strictures and when patients need a dilator for self-bougienage at home. Maloney dilators are usually 75 cm long and range in diameter of the shaft from 12 French Gauge (F) to 60F (3F = 1 mm.) There are no applications for the Hurst dilator today.

Tapered polyvinyl dilators. In 1955, Puestow described a revolutionary approach for management of esophageal stenoses. He described a method whereby a steel guidewire was inserted through the stenotic area and then a series of steel olives mounted onto a semiflexible carrier system were passed over the guidewire. For many years, this was the only dilating system with a guidewire available to gastrointestinal endoscopists. In 1980, Savary and Coll designed a new system comprised of a set of semiflexible tapered polyvinyl dilators with hollowed centers which could be threaded onto an endo-scopically inserted guidewire. Two types of tapered polyvinyl bougies are pictured in Figure 2.8.

The Savary dilators are similar to the Eder-Puestow dilators in principle but they are more logical in

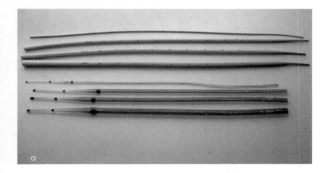

FIGURE 2.8 Tapered polyvinyl dilators. Products by two manufacturers displayed.

design. Increased flexibility make it easier to manipulate the dilators through the mouth. The "feel" of the dilator as it passes through the stricture is an important but subjective factor. Initially there was some concern that the polyvinyl dilators were not as readily apparent with fluoroscopy as the metal dilators, but either impregnation with barium—Bard® dilators—or the use of radiopaque markers on the dilator—Wilson-Cook® dilators—overcomes this problem.

Balloon dilators. Balloons made of polyethylene and other substances have been used for esophageal dilation of benign and malignant conditions as well as neuromuscular disorders. In the former instances, the balloons are smaller, generally in the range of 12 mm (36F) to 18 mm (54F). If the balloon is not too large, it can be passed through the biopsy channel of the endoscope and the dilation can occur under direct visualization (Fig. 2.9). In this situation a guidewire is not required. Alternatively, the balloon dilator can be passed over a guidewire and the procedure can be carried out with fluoroscopic control. When balloon dilators are utilized for achalasia, the latter balloon-guidewire setup is utilized. Many types of balloon dilators have been used for pneumatic dilation in the management of achalasia. Balloons are available with an inflation range from 30 mm (90F) to 50 mm (150F).

GUIDEWIRES
The use of guidewires throughout the digestive tract and pancreatico-biliary system is being employed with increasing frequency by gastrointestinal endoscopists and radiologists. It is likely that the newer generation of guidewires with hydrophilic coating(Glidewires®)and steering mechanisms will be utilized more frequently for difficult esophageal strictures in the near future. At present, the most commonly employed guidewire is one similar to that pictured in Figure 2.10. The guidewire itself is usually 200 cm in length with a wire diameter of 0.08 cm. Its distal spring tip is approximately 7 cm in length and 1.8 mm diameter. The wire is reinforced where it joins the spring tip so that it is unlikely to bend at this point. Guidewires with markings on them are available so that if the dilation is carried out without fluoroscopy, a reference point can be used.

ENDOSCOPES
When endoscopes are used to evaluate and treat dysphagia, in most instances standard 9 to 11 mm instruments can be used. However, it is wise to have a small 7.5 mm caliber instrument available in case there is a tight stenosis. It is expected that the smaller caliber miniscopes—1 to 5 mm—which are now experimental, will be useful in the future.

PROCEDURE

GENERAL PRINCIPLES
There are few contra-indications to esophageal dilation. Apart from a known esophageal perforation, the only other standard contra-indications are medical conditions which make the patient too unstable to be treated or a situation where the patient cannot cooperate and puts both himself and health personnel

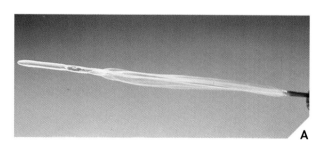
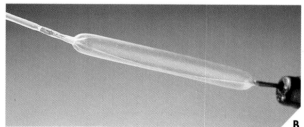

A

B

FIGURE 2.9 A through-the-scope balloon dilator is deflated when passed through the endoscope (**A**) and then inflated (**B**).

at risk. Relative contra-indications include severe cardiopulmonary disease, recent laparotomy, a large thoracic aneurysm, and a known bleeding disorder. If the patient is on an anticoagulant and it can be stopped prior to the dilation, that is a logical plan. If the clinical situation warrants dilation, however, patients with all of the relative contra-indications may be dilated. In patients with esophageal cancer, ongoing radiation therapy is not a contra-indication to dilation.

Informed consent should emphasize the potential complications which may occur and the patient should understand what the therapeutic plan will be if the complication does occur. This is also the ideal time to reassure the patient that esophageal dilation is safe. He should be told that breathing will be unaffected during the procedure and that he will be able to signal to you if there is a problem.

The patient should be kept NPO for at least 8 hr prior to the procedure. In patients in whom there is a high probability of esophageal retention of food or fluid, such as achalasia, consideration should be given to intubating the esophagus with a large bore tube to aspirate retained esophageal contents.

The physician should also ready himself prior to the procedure. It is useful to have the esophagram present for reference and if the patient has had a recent endoscopy, that report should be at hand. Check the equipment. If the rubber dilators show cracking, they should be replaced. Balloon dilators should be tested to make sure there are no leaks.

The risk of bacteremia with esophageal dilation has been the subject of several studies. In some studies, the incidence has been as high as 50%. Bacteremia is more common if the dilator is being passed through necrotic tissue. One study suggested that the instance of bacteremia could be reduced by disinfecting the dilators prior to the procedure. That is not the standard policy in my practice. Antibiotics should be strongly considered if the patient has a prosthetic heart valve or a previous history of endocarditis.

In many patients with known simple peptic strictures who have been dilated in the past, the procedure can be carried out with no intravenous sedation. The patient is in a sitting position and the only premedication is topical, oropharyngeal anesthesia with a xylocaine spray or gargle. If the procedure is to be carried out in conjunction with endoscopy, the patient is placed in the left lateral decubitus position and meperidine and a benzodiazepine are used for sedation. Midazolam is commonly employed. Anticholinergics are not used routinely.

If fluoroscopy is available in the endoscopy unit, it is generally used with esophageal dilation. Fluoroscopy is not available in many endoscopy units, which means that it will have to be performed in the radiology suite. Because this may involve some scheduling difficulties and may increase the cost of the procedure, the physician should determine in advance whether or not fluoroscopy is necessary for a given procedure. The variables that affect the need for fluoroscopy include the:

• Nature of the pathologic process.
• Possibility of an associated therapeutic procedure.

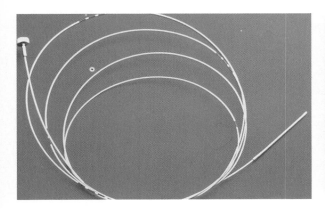 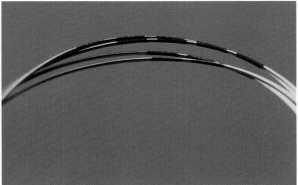

FIGURE 2.10 Guidewire used for esophageal dilation. It is flexible, has a spring tip, and impregnated markings.

- Endoscopic extent of the exam.
- Geography of the stricture.
- Experience of the endoscopist (Table 2.2).

Fluoroscopy is always required with certain pathological processes, such as esophageal diverticula, a large or para-esophageal hiatal hernia, a known fistula, or a previous perforation. For therapeutic procedures such as stent placement or pneumatic dilation with achalasia, fluoroscopy is always required.

Fluoroscopy may not be mandatory if dilation is performed for a simple peptic stricture, a web or ring, a corrosive stricture, radiation stricture, or for a post surgical anastomosis. In some malignant strictures, fluoroscopy is not always required for dilation. If fluoroscopy is not to be utilized, a previously obtained radiograph should demonstrate that the anatomy is not distorted. One is less apt to use fluoroscopy in the latter group of stenoses when an endoscope can be passed beyond the stricture.

The geography of the stricture may also influence the need for fluoroscopy. If an acute angle or previous surgery has distorted the anatomy, if the lumen is not obvious, if a fistula exists or if there are multiple sites of narrowing, fluoroscopy should always be utilized. Naturally, the experience of the physician performing the procedure enters into the final decision. It should be remembered that the patient's safety rather than the physician's convenience is the vital common pathway.

Before beginning the procedure, think about what type of dilators will be utilized. The decision about what size the first dilator should be is based on the observed luminal size if this is the first dilation for a particular patient. If it is a repeat dilation, some information can be gleaned from the previous procedure. If an endoscope has passed through the strictured area, I will usually begin with a dilator that is the same diameter as the endoscope. It is psychologically important for the patient to have the first dilation go smoothly. Small diameter Maloney dilators less than 30F tend to curl upon themselves and are of little use for most dilations. An important concept to appreciate is that not all of the dilation needs to occur in one sitting. It should be remembered that in almost all cases, the stricture formed over weeks or months rather than days and that an attempt to perform all the dilations in one sitting may increase the risk of perforation. Many

TABLE 2.2 VARIABLES AFFECTING THE NEED FOR FLUOROSCOPY WITH ESOPHAGEAL DILATION

Variable	Example(s) Where Fluoroscopy Should be Used
• Nature of pathologic process	Esophageal diverticula, paraesophageal hiatal hernia, known fistula
• Associated therapeutic procedure	Stent placement, achalasia
• Endoscopic extent of exam	Complicated anatomy and endoscope does not pass beyond stricture
• Geography of stricture narrowing	Acute angle, multiple sites, if lumen not obvious
• Experience of endoscopist	Physician with limited dilation experience

physicians follow the "rule of three" popularized by Dr. Boyce in terms of knowing how many dilators to use in a given setting. This rules states that dilation should end when resistance is encountered with three consecutive dilators. Only experience can teach how much resistance is significant, but for reasons mentioned above it is wiser to err on the conservative side. The finding of blood on a dilator after it is passed may or may not be important. If the stricture is friable and hemorrhagic prior to the procedure, it may be of little importance. Conversely, if the lesion was not bleeding prior to the procedure, it makes sense to consider the observation. There is no absolute endpoint to dilation in terms of diameter of the bougie, but if there is not significant resistance, dilation is carried out until a 42F or 45F instrument has been passed. During the procedure, one also tries to assess the texture of the stricture. If the stricture is fibrotic, part of the strategy is to fracture the stenosis. Often the physician will note the change from marked resistance to a more receptive passage. If the stricture is extremely elastic, graduated dilations seldom lead to improvement.

Is endoscopy necessary after dilation? If the stricture has prevented full endoscopic evaluation of the entire narrowed segment and the upper gastrointestinal tract has not been visualized, endoscopy should be performed. If the patient has not been previously dilated, it is reasonable to repeat the endoscopy after the procedure to notice what changes have occurred. Some bleeding is to be expected and the strictured area can appear raw with linear tears. If the patient has been dilated previously, routine endoscopy after the procedure is not necessary unless a specific question is to be addressed.

The patient should be observed for at least an hour after the procedure and written instructions are always given. Patients should be instructed to contact the physician if chest pain persists and particularly if it worsens. Hematemesis, shortness of breath, fever or patient concern are all reasons for which the physician should be contacted.

SPECIFIC TECHNIQUES

MALONEY DILATORS

A patient with a simple peptic stricture that has been endoscoped and dilated on a previous occasion might undergo the procedure without sedation. The patient should sit in a stable, four-legged chair with arm rests. The throat should be sprayed with a topical anesthetic. Dentures should be removed. The patient is reassured as above. The physician should wear a gown and be double-gloved. The patient is asked to flex his neck and open his mouth. If the physician is right-handed, he puts the index and middle fingers of his left hand toward the back of the patient's mouth. At this time, he tests the gag reflex to make sure that the throat is numbed. With his right hand he holds both the tip of the dilator and the string at the untapered end which is looped around the little finger on the right hand. This prevents the weight of the dilator from dragging towards the floor and making the passage more difficult.

The tip of the dilator is then advanced over the tongue and in between the two fingers that have been positioned at the back of the throat. The fingers in the mouth are used to guide the tip of the dilator posteriorly and inferiorly through the upper esophageal sphincter. When the tip of the dilator reaches the sphincter, the patient is asked to swallow. Additionally, the two fingers grab the dilator to prevent it from falling back out of the mouth. This allows the physician's right hand to slip down on the shaft to grab the dilator approximately 10 cm away from the incisors so that it can be advanced. If there is profound gagging, the dilator should be withdrawn but usually the patient can be reassured and the dilator easily advanced. Once the dilator is beyond the upper sphincter, it should be advanced in a steady, continuous motion. The physician takes note of the amount of resistance as the dilator is being advanced and once the shaft of the dilator has passed the stricture, it should be removed expediently. There is no advantage to leaving the dilator in the stricture once it has been passed. This procedure is continued, relying on the principles above to determine when the procedure should be ended (Fig. 2.11).

If the Maloney dilation is to occur after an endoscopic procedure or if it is done in a patient who requires sedation, it should be performed in the left lateral decubitus position. Although the patient is reclining, the hand positions and passage is performed in a similar manner as when the patient is sitting. A nurse should be available to suction secretions from the patient's mouth since he has been sedated. If fluoroscopy is being utilized, the passage of each dilator should be confirmed radiographically. If fluoroscopy is not being used, an experienced endoscopist can generally determine if the bougie is properly placed and whether it is advancing beyond the stricture. Excessive coughing and the inability to speak should raise concern that the dilator is in the trachea. If the dilator kinks or buckles at the patient's mouth, there should be concern that it is not advancing beyond the narrowed segment.

TAPERED POLYVINYL DILATORS

The technique for esophageal dilation requiring a guidewire is as follows. A small caliber endoscope is advanced to the area of the esophageal stenosis and, if at all possible, through the obstruction and into the stomach. This allows for full definition of the length and geography of the stenosis. After a screening endoscopy is completed, the endoscope is taken to the distal body or antrum. In the unoperated gastrointestinal (GI) tract, 60 cm usually represents the level of the distal body or antrum (refer to Fig. 4.8). The guidewire is then advanced through the biopsy channel beyond the distal tip of the scope. The endoscope is then withdrawn making sure that the guidewire does not slip from this spot. This is accomplished by alternately advancing the guidewire approximately 10 cm through the channel as the endoscope is withdrawn a like distance. This allows the guidewire to remain where it was placed in the antrum. After the endoscope is removed, the endoscopist then checks the marks on the guidewire.

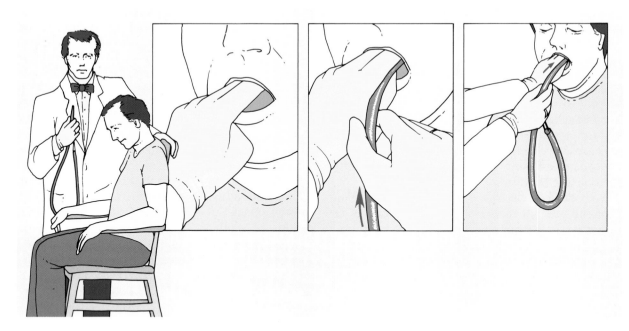

FIGURE 2.11 Bougienage with Maloney dilators without sedation. Right-handed physician stands to the right of the patient who is seated in the chair with neck flexed. Index and middle fingers of the left hand depress the posterior area of the tongue and serve to guide the dilator in midline to the pharynx. Dilation proceeds with advancement of the bougie using the right hand.

Each mark represents a distance of 20 cm. If there are 3 markings on the wire at the incisors, the tip of the guidewire will be 60 cm distally.

The technique for guidewire placement, if the small-caliber endoscope cannot be advanced beyond the stenosis, is as follows. With the endoscope at the proximal margin of the stenosis, the guidewire is advanced through the endoscopic channel and then into the stricture. The endoscopist should know from a previous contrast study of the upper GI tract that passage beyond the stenotic area will not lead the guidewire into any unusually sharp angulations or crevices. If the upper GI x-ray suggests that this is the case, then the procedure should not be done without fluoroscopic observation. If the passageway beyond the stenosis appears to be relatively straight, the guidewire is advanced. Generally, no significant resistance is encountered. If there is resistance, the endoscopic procedure should be done only with fluoroscopic control. However, if the guidewire advances easily, it should be passed beyond the stenosis for approximately 20 to 40 more cm. This will carry the wire into position in the distal body or proximal antrum. The same technique is used for withdrawing the endoscope and advancing the guidewire. Again, in the unoperated stomach, it should be left with 3 markings at the incisors (60 cm). After the guidewire has been properly positioned, either with or without direct visualization, progressively larger dilators can be passed.

Some physicians use a guidewire and fluoroscope to pass tapered polyvinyl dilators without employing an endoscope. With this technique, the guidewire is passed as if it were using the same principles as a Maloney dilator. Fluoroscopic monitoring is required. If the guidewire gets hung up at the stricture, the physician can maneuver it by flipping the coil of wire which is held in his hand outside the patient's mouth. Torque will be transferred along the course of the wire and it generally falls into proper position.

BALLOON DILATORS

As mentioned previously, balloon dilators may be either used through the endoscope without a guidewire or they may be passed over a guidewire. Smaller balloon sizes are used for esophageal strictures and larger balloons used over a guidewire for the management of achalasia. The balloon can be filled with either air, water, or contrast material. Manometers or pressure gauges are usually supplied by the manufacturer with specific instructions as to what pressure is acceptable for a given balloon. There is no evidence that filling the balloon with either contrast or water conveys a substantial benefit. If contrast material is utilized, it is usually diluted 1:4 with saline. This allows it to be visualized fluoroscopically. With the dilution, the material becomes less viscous and it is easier to fill the balloon. The end point of dilation, when the balloon is passed via the scope, is when the waist at the proximal margin of the stricture appears to be lost and the stricture takes on the same diameter as the balloon. If the stricture is ruptured, there is generally a sudden fall in pressure on the gauge signifying that the stricture has been dilated. If the procedure is carried out with fluoroscopic control, it is deemed successful when the waist which had been seen in the balloon fluoroscopically is lost. Once the balloon is fully dilated, there is no consensus as to how long balloon expansion should be maintained. Thirty seconds is common.

When the through the scope method of balloon dilation is employed, a large channel therapeutic endoscope is chosen. A collapsed 12 mm (36F) balloon catheter can pass through a 3.5 mm channel. After the patient is sedated, the endoscope is advanced to the proximal margin of the stricture. The assistant exerts negative pressure on the balloon as the endoscopist advances it beyond the distal end of the endoscope and into the stricture. The balloons come in different lengths and diameters. Based on the radiographic appearance of the stricture, a balloon of a given length will be chosen. It is advanced from the endoscope and into the stricture. The endoscopist will observe the superior portion of the balloon as it is being inflated. A waist is generally observed. The assistant will be monitoring the pressure so that the balloon can be inflated to the appropriate level. As mentioned above, the balloon will remain inflated for 30 sec at this pressure or until there is a sudden drop in the manometric reading. With successful dilation, the waist is obliterated. Some blood may be noted on the balloon as it is withdrawn. After the dilation has been carried out, it may be possible to pass the large diameter endoscope through the stricture, but in most cases it is not and then a small caliber endoscope will be used.

When balloon dilation is carried out over a guidewire, fluoroscopy must be used. The guidewire is passed by advancing the endoscope to the proximal margin of the stricture as previously described with polyvinyl dilators. The guidewire is observed and positioned fluoroscopically. The endoscope is then removed and the balloon catheter is advanced over the guidewire. The appropriate length of the balloon will be chosen. Over the wire, balloons up to 20 mm (60F) can be utilized. Radiopaque markers define the proximal and distal extent of the balloon. The balloon should be centered in the stricture. Usually an attempt is made to dilate the stricture to 45F. Patient discomfort may be a limitation to reaching that goal.

PNEUMATIC DILATION FOR ACHALASIA

The actual technique for pneumatic or hydrostatic dilation for achalasia is very similar to over the guidewire dilation for esophageal strictures. The goal of the forceful dilation is to tear circular muscle and to effect lasting reduction in lower esophageal sphincter pressure. To minimize the risk of aspiration or contamination if a perforation were to occur, it is important to clear the esophagus of fluid and food debris before performing the procedure. To accomplish this, the patient is kept on a clear liquid diet for 24 to 48 hrs prior to the procedure. In addition, if there is retained material a large bore (34F) evacuation tube should be passed and debris be removed with suction. A baseline chest x-ray is obtained as well as blood work to check coagulation parameters and hematocrit. Blood is typed and screened as an additional precaution. It is wise to notify a thoracic surgeon that the procedure is being performed, in case a perforation occurs.

On rare occasions, patients with long-standing achalasia have a fibrotic stricture. Therefore, it is useful to screen for such a finding, because if it is found, pneumatic dilation can be avoided. In such patients, pass a single 54F Maloney dilator. With classic achalasia, the dilator passes easily through the lower sphincter. If there is a fibrotic stricture, distinct resistance will be met. If so, the pneumatic dilation is not performed and the patient is evaluated clinically and/or radiographically to see if benefit is realized.

If no stricture is found, standard balloon dilation for achalasia can be performed with fluoroscopic guidance. The patient is placed in the left lateral decubitis position and the guidewire is placed. The

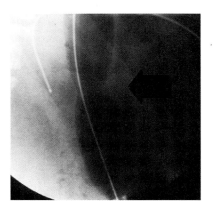 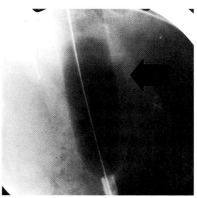

FIGURE 2.12 Radiograph showing balloon dilation for achalasia. Initially, the balloon is inflated and a waist at the region of the lower esophageal sphincter is noted. The goal of the dilation is to obliterate the waist which usually correlates with a successful procedure. (Courtesy of Dr. Stanley Benjamin)

position is confirmed fluoroscopically. The balloon is usually expanded with air, although in some cases saline or contrast material is used (Fig. 2.12).

The most common balloon dilators used for achalasia are 30, 35 and 40 mm. It is standard practice to begin with the 30 mm balloon dilator. Under fluoroscopic control, the balloon is positioned so that its midsection is at the high pressure segment (Fig. 2.13A). There is considerable variation among physicians regarding some specifics of the procedure. There is debate as to how rapidly the balloon should be inflated, whether the end point should be a given pressure or obliteration of the waist, and how long the balloon should stay dilated. A recent study suggested that there was no difference in efficacy or safety when the balloon was inflated until waist obliteration or inflated to a given pressure and held for 2 minutes. The technique I have followed is to inflate the balloon until the waist is obliterated and to maintain inflation for 1 minute after the waist is gone. The procedure is shown schematically in Fig. 2.13. The patient may experience some pain when the balloon is fully dilated and some blood is often seen when the dilator is removed.

My own policy is to admit the patient for overnight observation after the procedure although recently there have been some reports describing the performance of the procedure as an out-patient. A chest x-ray is performed immediately after the procedure to look for free air. My own policy is to perform a water soluble contrast esophagram the next

morning after maintaining the patient NPO. Alternatively, the esophagram can be performed after the patient is fully awake. If there are no complications, a normal diet may be started on the day following the procedure.

An easy and objective means of assessing the efficacy of the pneumatic dilation—in addition to the patient's symptoms—is to compare the height of a standing column of barium with the patient in an upright position. An oblique film is taken and the height of the column in centimeters is recorded (Fig. 2.14). Comparisons are made between radiographs taken before the dilation and at least 4 weeks after the procedure.

Self-Bougienage

It is uncommon in most physicians' practices to encounter a large number of patients for whom self-bougienage will be appropriate, but on occasion it is desirable. The patient must be confident, well-motivated, and intelligent enough to understand basic medical principles and anatomy. It may be particularly useful if a patient lives in a remote area or has difficulty getting to a medical facility. It should only be used for simple, benign strictures.

Preparation for the patient involves a didactic explanation of the relevant anatomy, the esophagram, technique and possible complications. Pictures or models showing the relationship of the pharynx, larynx, and esophagus should be used. It is useful for

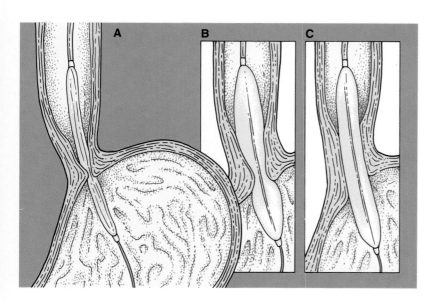

Figure 2.13 Technique for pneumatic dilation for achalasia. Under fluoroscopic control, the balloon is positioned so that its midsection is at the high pressure segment **(A)**. The balloon is inflated and the endoscopist observes a waist seen fluoroscopically **(B)**. With successful dilation, the waist is obliterated **(C)**.

the patient to see his own esophagram. A discussion of the signs and symptoms of potential complications should be reviewed.

Often fear is the most important difficulty for the patient to overcome. This can be addressed by having the first several self-dilations be performed with the physician present. It is also useful for the patient to speak with other patients who have done self-bougienage.

Usually the patient will utilize a single Maloney dilator— 42F/44F or 46F. It should be marked with indelible ink at 20 cm from its tapered end and at a point 10 cm beyond the stricture (Fig. 2.15). When given the choice, most patients do not wish to apply a topical anesthetic prior to dilation. The patient is in a sitting position.

After the dilator is lubricated with water, the tapered end is introduced over the tongue with the left hand. The index finger guides the tip to the back of the throat. At the beginning of the procedure, the other end of the dilator hangs down in the patient's lap and is held by the patient's right hand. When the tip of the dilator encounters the region of the upper esophageal sphincter, the patient swallows, and the dilator is advanced with the right hand. When the patient sees the first marking at 20 cm, he assumes, if he is not choking, that the dilator has reached the esophagus. He then raises the tip of the dilator held in his right hand straight up above his head. This allows the mercury to migrate to the tapered end. Then pushing slowly with the right hand and using the left to guide, the dilator is advanced through the stenosis. The patient knows he has advanced it enough when he sees the second ink marking reach lip level. The technique is illustrated in Figure 2.16.

MANAGEMENT OF SPECIFIC TYPES OF STRICTURES

PEPTIC STRICTURES

Maloney dilators, balloons, or tapered-polyvinyl dilators are all useful for most peptic strictures. There is no convincing data suggesting that one is safer or more efficacious than another. The patient will usually determine the frequency with which dilation is carried out. They have an uncanny knack for balancing the dissimilar displeasures of dysphagia and dilation. Although a tradition of performing the procedure without sedation has evolved, I personally prefer to sedate patients even for this "simple procedure." I

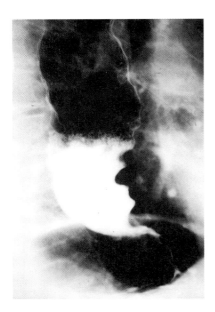

FIGURE 2.14 Esophagram in a patient with achalasia. The standing column of barium measures 7 cm in height prior to pneumatic dilation.

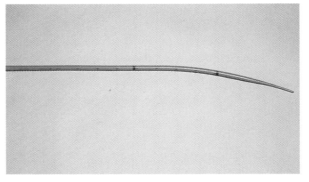

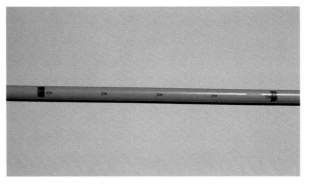

FIGURE 2.15 Dilator marked at point 20 cm from distal tip and at 42 cm, a point 10 cm beyond the location of the stricture, which was 32 cm from the incisors.

believe the lack of discomfort and relative amnesia outweigh the purported disadvantages of added expense and postprocedure observation time. If the patient dreads the thought of being dilated, they are less apt to return when symptoms first reappear. Treatment with omeprazole or H_2-antagonists in doses high enough to suppress acid reflux are important components of therapy and tend to lengthen the span between subsequent dilations.

CORROSIVE INJURIES

Maloney or tapered polyvinyl dilators are used when dilation for acute corrosive injuries is required. If the injury is circumferential a stricture can be anticipated. It is necessary to individualize the timing for complicated third-degree injuries. Once the patient is stable and it is determined that there is no extra-esophageal injury or perforation, early dilation is recommended. Stricturing usually occurs by the third week, so dilation should be undertaken by at least one week following the injury.

For dilation of chronic, long standing corrosive strictures, extreme caution is needed. Even though the esophageal lumen may be only a few mm wide, the patient often has learned to compensate with prolonged mastication and lubrication. Dilation should be extremely gradual and may require five or more sessions. There is no rush to open the lumen. The physician should appreciate that an advance from 5 to 8 mm represents an improvement of more than 50%. Dilation should be performed every 2 to 3 weeks. One generally begins with either the last dilator used at the previous session or even the next to last size. These strictures are often long and if they can be dilated to 10 or 11 mm, patients will note tremendous improvement.

POSTRADIATION STRICTURES

These strictures may be long and very firm so tapered polyvinyl dilators should be employed. It is also useful to dilate gradually reaching maximum diameter after 2 to 4 sessions. Repeated dilations may be necessary.

POSTSCLEROTHERAPY STRICTURES

Most often postsclerotherapy dysphagia is caused by stricture formation from the sclerosant itself, although other mechanisms have been postulated. Some

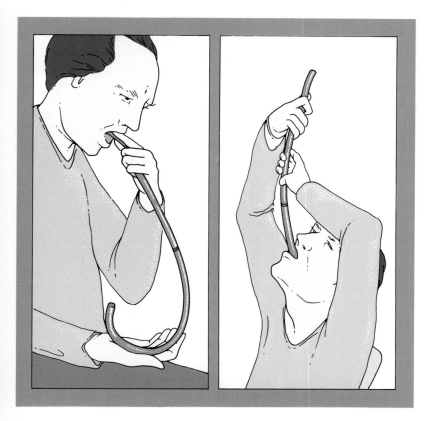

FIGURE 2.16 Technique of self-bougienage. In the seated position, the tapered end of the dilator is introduced over the tongue with the left hand. The index finger guides the tip to the back of the throat. When the tip of the dilator encounters the region of the upper esophageal sphincter, the patient swallows and the dilator is advanced with the right hand. Once the patient sees the first marking at 20 cm, he assumes that he has reached the esophagus. The dilator is then steadily advanced through the stenosis.

manometric evidence supports the development of motility disorders postprocedure and there are isolated reports of increased reflux after sclerosis. For stricturing due to scleroscent-induced injury, dilation with Maloney dilators, balloons, and tapered polyvinyl dilators have been effective. There are no comparative studies in this subgroup.

TUMOR PROBE THERAPY STRICTURES
Dilation of strictures caused by localized circumferential thermal injury can be more difficult than dilations of the original neoplasm. These strictures are extremely fibrotic. With these stenoses, tapered polyvinyl dilators alone are useful. It is necessary to perform endoscopy after dilation to make certain that the narrowed segment was actually fractured. Anecdotal experience with steroid injection into the stricture to delay reformation has not proved uniformly beneficial.

PILL-INDUCED
Once the proper diagnosis is established, the most important aspect of therapy is to discontinue the offending agent. If strictures develop, they are usually localized but may be very fibrotic. Tapered polyvinyl dilators are preferred.

SCHATZKI'S RING
Since the goal of therapy is rupture of the ring, dilation with a single large Maloney or polyvinyl dilator has been the conventional approach rather than standard progressive stretching. Therefore, the initial dilation should be carried out with at least a 50F dilator. For many years, it was the teaching that a single dilation lasted a lifetime. Recent prospective data has shown that repeated dilation is required. In one series, only two thirds of patients were dysphagia free at 1 year and only 10% of patients had no recurrent symptoms at 5 years. Since there appears to be a decreased frequency of reflux in patients with Schatzki's ring, suppression of acid reflux is not a component of therapy.

MALIGNANT STRICTURES
Tapered polyvinyl dilators are clearly the bougies of choice for malignant stenoses. Since the benefit of dilating malignant strictures is short-lived, dilation is often performed in concert with another therapy (refer to Chapter 4). The endoscopist must be particularly wary of false channels and fluoroscopic imaging may be necessary. When dilation precedes laser or tumor probe therapy, the goal is often to open the lumen so that therapy can begin at the distal tumor margin. When a stent is required for treatment of esophageal cancer, I prefer to perform the dilation in at least 2 sessions unless there is a fistula for which emergency placement is required. This allows for gradual stretching and the insertion on the second day generally goes more smoothly. Additionally, the endoscopist can take precise measurements at the time of the first dilation so that the proper stent can be chosen and all the equipment made ready in advance.

COMPLICATIONS

PERFORATIONS
The most serious complication of esophageal dilation is perforation. The reported incidence is approximately 1:500 dilations. The variables listed in Table 2.2 which increase the need for fluoroscopy also increase the likelihood of perforation.

Pain is the most common symptom and may be accompanied by crepitus and fever. Free air in the chest or abdomen may accompany the pain. It is not uncommon for a patient to have chest or throat discomfort after a difficult dilation but the clue is that the pain increases rather than decreases with time.

If there is any question, a contrast radiograph must be obtained. It is generally accepted that radiographic evaluation should begin with a water-soluble contrast agent followed by barium esophagography if no extravasation is seen. However, in patients at risk for aspiration or in whom an esophago-respiratory fistula is expected, hypertonic water-soluble contrast agents such as gastrograffin are contraindicated since entrance into the lungs may cause pulmonary edema. Recently a low-osmolality water-soluble iodinated agent, iohexol, has become available and is advantageous in cases of esophageal disruption.

The nature of the perforation related to dilation is variable. With Maloney dilators, the perforation is usually proximal to the stricture. With balloon dilators, it usually occurs at the site of the stretching. Guidewires may cause perforation by creating a false channel outside the esophageal lumen over which the dilator is passed. Rarely, and more commonly with older guidewires that were not reinforced at the juncture of the spring tip and wire, the guidewire would kink, forming a sharp lead point and causing perforation (Fig. 2.17). There is no evidence that mucosal biopsies taken at endoscopy prior to actual dilation, increase the likelihood of a perforation.

The management of esophageal perforation following dilation depends upon the setting in which it occurs. If perforation follows pneumatic dilation for achalasia in a patient who has been properly prepared and whose esophagus has been evacuated, immediate surgery can be carried out if the leak is recognized early. Exploration, drainage, a Heller myotomy, and closure of the tear can be performed simultaneously. Alternatively, if a perforation follows dilation of a malignant esophageal stricture, medical management is preferred. A nasogastric tube is placed for aspiration above the tumor and antibiotics are begun. Analgesics are usually required for pain. If the long term prognosis justifies it, parenteral nutrition may be begun. For perforation following dilation of simple peptic strictures, exploration and drainage is usually required. If the perforation is discovered and surgery is carried out within 24 hrs, then primary closure is usually performed.

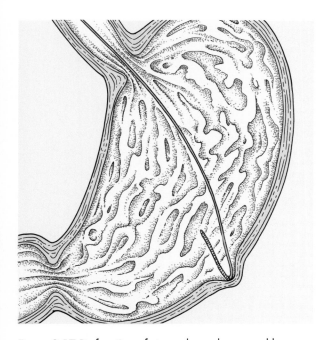

FIGURE 2.17 Perforation of stomach maybe caused by guidewire. Note bend at juncture of spring tip and wire which has indented the gastric wall.

BACTEREMIA

The incidence of bacteremia following esophageal dilation has ranged from 0% to more than 50%. It can be reduced by disinfecting the instruments prior to dilation. The incidence is greatest when necrotic or malignant tissue is traumatized. The most practical implication is that antibiotic prophylaxis should be employed in patients with prosthetic heart valves or a previous history of endocarditis and in patients who are severely immunocompromised.

OTHERS

Significant bleeding is extremely uncommon and massive hemorrhage is seen only with pneumatic dilation for achalasia. With malignant strictures, dilation can trigger arrhythmias, particularly if there is pericardial involvement. The physician should note that dilation of cancers residing in the upper esophagus can precipitate bronchospasm. Aspiration is rare and the importance of clearing the esophagus prior to dilation for achalasia has been emphasized.

Tooth dislodgement can occur any time instruments traverse the mouth. A sore throat is not uncommon after dilation, but it seldom is problematic. A warning prior to the procedure that it is to be anticipated and a lozenge following the procedure go a long way.

REFERENCES

Dumon JF, Meric B, Sivak MV, Fleischer DE. A new method of esophageal dilation using Savary-Gilliard bougies. *Gastrointest Endosc* 1985;31:379.

Earlam R and Cunha-Melo: Benign oesophageal strictures: Historical and technical aspects of dilation. *Br J Surg* 1981;68:829.

Esophageal dilation. Guidelines for clinical application. *Gastrointest Endosc* 1991. (In press).

Tulman AB and Boyce HW: Complications of esophageal dilation and guidelines for their prevention. *Gastrointest Endosc* 1981;27:229.

Webb WA: Esophageal dilation: Personal experience with current instruments and techniques. *Am J Gastroenterol* 1988;83:471.

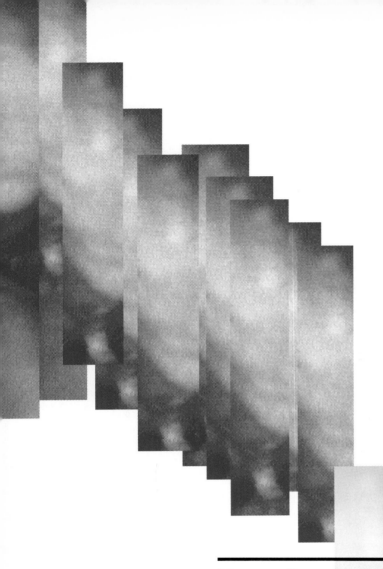

Esophageal Variceal Sclerotherapy

3

Jerome D. Waye, MD

INTRODUCTION

Acute hemorrhage from esophageal varices is a common clinical problem with high morbidity and mortality despite medical or surgical treatment (Fig. 3.1). Interest in esophageal variceal sclerotherapy, a technique first described over 40 years ago, has been rekindled because of disappointing results in controlled trials of shunt surgery for bleeding esophageal varices.

Flexible endoscopes enable accurate identification of the source of upper gastrointestinal hemorrhage. The trained endoscopist now has the additional capability of a treatment option once the diagnosis of esophageal variceal bleeding has been confirmed (Fig. 3.2). Esophageal variceal sclerotherapy (EVS) is a technique which is more effective than standard medical therapy and is at least as effective as surgery in controlling both acute and recurrent variceal hemorrhage. The technique is detailed in this chapter.

INDICATIONS

Currently the most common indication for EVS is the cessation and prevention of recurrent bleeding in

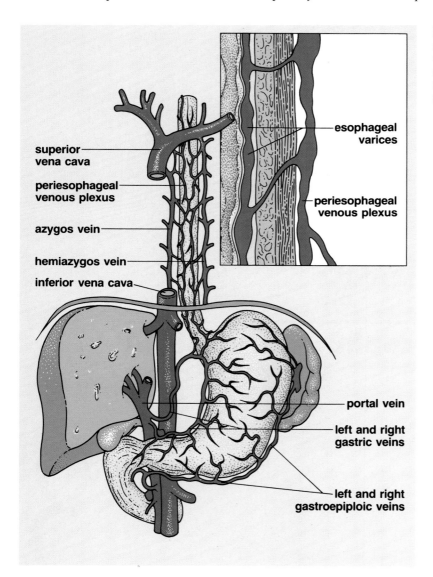

FIGURE 3.1 Schematic diagram of the normal venous system. Esophageal varices result from portal hypertension. Insert shows the interconnection of esophageal varices and periesophageal venous plexus.

esophageal varices

periesophageal venous plexus

superior vena cava

periesophageal venous plexus

azygos vein

hemiazygos vein

inferior vena cava

portal vein

left and right gastric veins

left and right gastroepiploic veins

patients who have had at least one episode of major gastrointestinal hemorrhage caused by esophageal varices.

Endoscopic sclerotherapy has the capability of stopping acute variceal hemorrhage in over 90% of the patients in whom it is used. Currently, the accepted practice is to perform sclerotherapy of varices during the emergency endoscopic examination. Balloon tamponade with a Sengstaken-Blakemore tube to control massive hemorrhage is rarely used.

There is controversy as to the appropriateness of prophylactic sclerotherapy to obliterate varices that have never bled.

PATIENT ASSESSMENT

One problem in assessing patient eligibility for endoscopic sclerotherapy is in determining whether a particular bleeding episode was indeed caused by esophageal varices rather than by some other pathology. Prior to undertaking any EVS treatment, a complete endoscopic examination of the esophagus, stomach, and duodenum is performed. Frequently active blood loss has stopped and no bleeding lesion can be identified during this initial endoscopy. The endoscopist must seek the presence of a duodenal or gastric ulceration, Mallory-Weiss laceration, gastritis, or the presence of any other lesion that could have caused hemorrhage. In the absence of any other potential bleeding sites such as these, the finding of esophageal varices in the patient who recently bled is sufficient evidence to implicate the varices as the cause of bleeding. Injection sclerotherapy should be carried out only after other possibilities are eliminated.

EVS is an important alternative for poor surgical candidates, although it has rapidly become the treatment of choice even for good surgical risks.

EQUIPMENT

Several techniques have been utilized for EVS. Rigid or flexible fiberoptic instruments with general anesthesia, or flexible endoscopes with intravenous sedation or without any medication are the primary modalities. It has been suggested that fiberoptic scopes be modified with a semirigid overtube, fitted with an inflatable balloon cuff, or utilized with a balloon inflated in the cardia of the stomach.

Proponents of rigid endoscopy state that bleeding from a variceal puncture site can be easily controlled by compression with the metal tube. Some rigid endoscopes have been modified with a notch on the distal-most end to permit a varix to bulge into the lumen facilitating its fixation for injection. There is little to recommend rigid endoscopy today except that surgeons familiar with this technique continue to use it. An innovative overtube is available for the fiberoptic instrument with a longitudinal "slot" in its distal end. When preloaded onto the endoscope, it may be slid into the esophagus beyond the endoscope tip, causing a varix to bulge into the slot. Rotation of the overtube after injection provides tamponade. In general, gastroenterologists prefer the flexible instruments without an overtube, performing injections with a retractable needle passed through the instrument channel.

Some endoscopists attempt to decrease the blood flow rate in esophageal varices prior to EVS, and use traction on an inflatable balloon in the stomach fun-

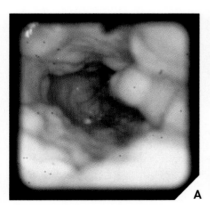 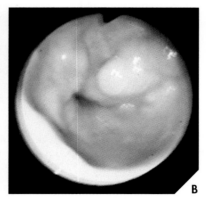

FIGURE 3.2 Esophageal varices are readily identified endoscopically, and may be extensive (**A**) or relatively discrete (**B**).

dus. Others prefer an inflatable balloon cuff on the endoscope to impede cephalad variceal blood flow, distending the varices for easier injection. The cuff may also be used to tamponade the bleeding site. There is little evidence, however, that any of these devices is better than sclerotherapy performed with a "freehand" technique.

SCLEROSANTS

Several solutions are available for sclerotherapy, and the technique of sclerotherapy is dependent to some extent on the type of solution available. In the United States, the three agents most commonly employed are sodium morrhuate (5% solution), sodium tetradecyl-sulfate (STS) (1% or 3% solution), and ethanolamine oleate. In Europe there is a preference for ethanolamine oleate or polidocanol (Aethoxysklerol).

All the solutions may be given directly into or around the esophageal varices with the exception of polidocanol, which should not be administered intra-venously and is usually injected into the paravariceal tissue. Sodium morrhuate and sodium tetradecylsulfate may be injected in 1 to 5 mL increments. Whether the endoscopist intends to administer an agent directly into the varix lumen may be academic since evidence exists that when attempting to inject a sclerosant solution directly into a varix the substance actually is deposited in the wall of the esophagus (paravariceal) 40% of the time. Since inadvertent paravariceal injections are so commonly given and difficult to avoid, many sclerotherapists purposely utilize a combination of intra and paravariceal injections (Fig. 3.3).

FREEHAND TECHNIQUE

The freehand technique for endoscopic sclerotherapy is the most preferred procedure. The entire injection sclerotherapy session consists of 5 to 20 separate

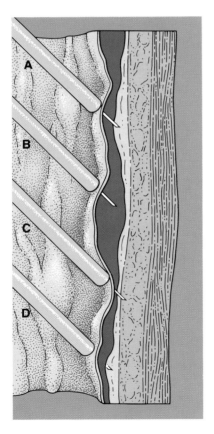

FIGURE 3.3 Although the intended sites for injection of sclerosant solution are intravariceal, injections are deposited frequently into paravariceal areas. Injection through the vein to the submucosa. (A) Injection directly into a bulging varix. (B) Injection into the muscular layer of the wall. (C) Injection into paravariceal tissues missing the varix (D).

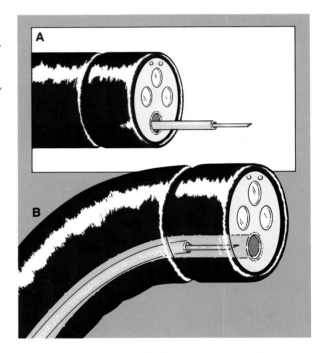

FIGURE 3.4 Once the needle has been extended from its protective sheath (A), there is no need to retract it into the sheath again. The esophagus is protected from any injury that might result from sudden movement of the patient by withdrawing the sheath and extended needle into the biopsy/suction channel (B).

esophageal needle punctures each delivering 1 to 4 mL of solution over the course of about 5 to 15 min. The total amount of sclerosant is about 20 mL.

Following a thorough examination of the stomach and duodenum, place the endoscope tip in the fundus of the stomach. The sheathed injection needle is passed through the biopsy port and flushed with the desired solution. Once the needle is extended from its sheath it is not necessary to retract it again. The esophagus may be safely protected by withdrawal of the entire catheter and needle into the endoscope's accessory channel so that the needle tip does not protrude beyond the end of the gastroscope (Fig. 3.4). The sheath is always held by the right hand whenever the needle tip is unprotected as it protrudes beyond the gastroscope: This permits immediate withdrawal of the sharp needle tip if the patient retches, coughs or belches air.

With the patient lying in the left lateral position, the endoscope, with the needle tip lying completely within the channel, is withdrawn from the stomach into the distal-most esophagus. Air is liberally insufflated during endoscopic sclerotherapy to distend the esophageal lumen, permitting adequate visualization.

In the absence of active bleeding, the sites for the first few injections should be carefully chosen, since blood tends to pool on the left wall of the esophagus during this technique. Therefore, the first injections should be directed toward the left wall of the distal-most esophagus because bleeding may soon obscure vision of that area (Fig. 3.5).

The tip of the endoscope is positioned 1 to 3 cm from the wall of the esophagus and the sheath is advanced by the right hand. Once the needle tip is visualized, the endoscopist maneuvers it toward the intended site of injection by rotating his body while the left thumb provides fine tip motion adjustment by moving the up/down control knob. Once in position, the needle is thrust directly into the desired site by rapidly advancing the sheath, plunging the needle

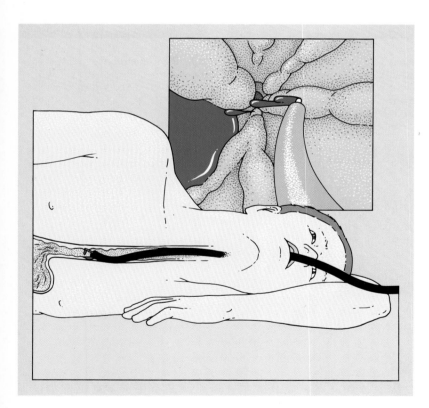

FIGURE 3.5 With the patient lying in the left lateral position, any blood from injection sites will pool on the left (dependent) wall, obscuring the view of that wall. Injections should commence, therefore, on the left wall and proceed clockwise or counter-clockwise. Inset shows blood collecting on the left wall which is at the 9 o'clock position as viewed by the endoscopist.

into the wall up to its junction with the sheath (Figs. 3.6, 3.7). A 23 gauge sclerotherapy needle not longer than 5 mm in length will guard against complete penetration of the wall of the esophagus, or delivery of sclerosing solution deep into the esophageal wall where mediastinitis may ensue.

As soon as penetration has been achieved, the endoscopist instructs the gastrointestinal assistant to rapidly administer the chosen volume of sclerosant–1 to 4 mL. Immediately following delivery the assistant says "stop." The declaration "stop" may be the only signal that the injection has been completed because clinical signs such as a bulge of the wall, blanching of tissue, or distention of an injected vein may or may not be apparent (Fig. 3.8). As soon as the injection is given, the needle is withdrawn and rapidly reinserted into an adjacent site. Multiple injections may be given first into the dependent (left) wall, after which atten-

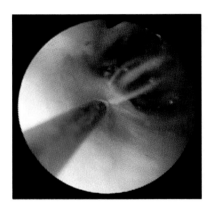

FIGURE 3.6 The injector needle is advanced to the hilt into a varix. During injection, some of the sclerosant solution may spill out of the injection site along the needle tract, as seen here.

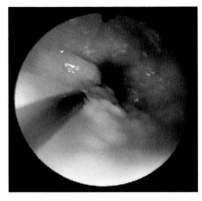

FIGURE 3.7 The injector needle has been placed beside a small varix to give a paravariceal injection. The raised mound at the 10 o'clock position is a pseudopolyp from previous sclerotherapy sessions.

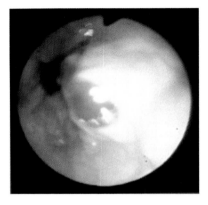

FIGURE 3.8 Appearance of a vein following intravariceal injection. The varix is swollen and slightly bleeding.

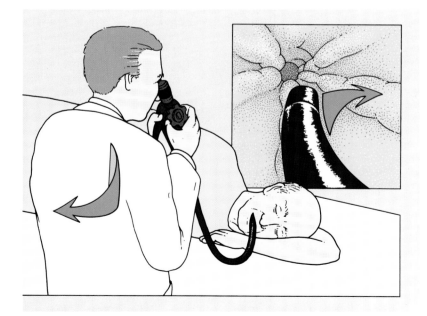

FIGURE 3.9 Because the endoscope is straight while in the esophagus, rotation of the endoscopist's body to the right will result in a corresponding rotation of the scope tip to the right. Any degree of tip deflection *(inset)* will further aid in maneuvering the endoscope toward the varices for injection of the right wall.

tion is directed toward the remainder of the esophagus, fully withdrawing the needle into the endoscope after each injection.

Maneuver the needle into position for injecting the right wall by a combination of tip deflection using the up/down control knob and torquing the instrument by rotating the endoscopist's body to the right. Initial injections to the left wall are delivered with the endoscopist's shoulders parallel to the axis of the esophagus; rotating the endoscopist's right shoulder away from the patient will permit the endoscope tip to swing toward the right wall of the esophagus (Fig. 3.9).

Multiple rapid injections are given circumferentially around the esophagus always beginning with the left wall. The site for the first injection should be just above the cardioesophageal mucosal junction. At this level, 4 or 6 multiple intra- and paravariceal injections may be given. The endoscope may then be withdrawn approximately 2 to 5 cm and circumferential injections given once again starting at the left wall and moving clockwise or counterclockwise around the esophageal circumference (Fig. 3.10).

The intravenously injected solution will travel cephalad, caudad, and into the veins draining the esophagus toward the lungs and toward the spinal column posteriorly. Blood mixes with the sclerosant solution as it leaves the esophageal varix, diluting its toxic effect before it circulates more than a few centimeters (Fig. 3.11). Refrain from intravariceal injections more proximally than 30 cm from the incisor

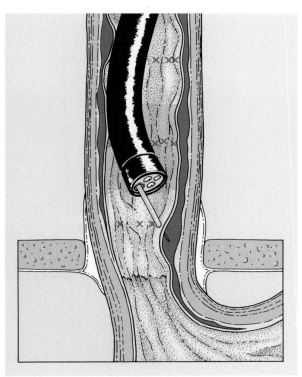

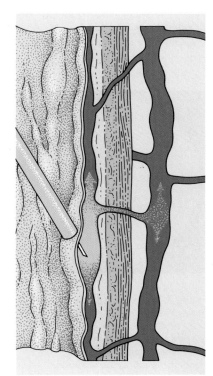

FIGURE 3.11 Following intravariceal injections, the sclerosant solution is rapidly diluted by blood. Most of it flows cephalad, a small amount flows retrograde into the varix, and the remainder is swept into the periesophageal venous plexus.

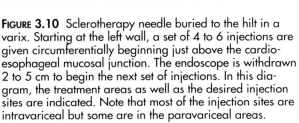

FIGURE 3.10 Sclerotherapy needle buried to the hilt in a varix. Starting at the left wall, a set of 4 to 6 injections are given circumferentially beginning just above the cardioesophageal mucosal junction. The endoscope is withdrawn 2 to 5 cm to begin the next set of injections. In this diagram, the treatment areas as well as the desired injection sites are indicated. Note that most of the injection sites are intravariceal but some are in the paravariceal areas.

teeth to guard against the possibility of undiluted sclerosant solution traveling to the spinal cord area where serious complications may ensue.

After each set of ten 1 mL injections, the endoscope is advanced into the stomach so that the lens may be cleansed with water and suction. Although most accessories occlude the suction/biopsy channel in the standard endoscope, the small diameter of most sclerotherapy sheaths permits some suction while the sclerotherapy needle is in place. Some endoscopists prefer a therapeutic instrument with a large accessory channel or with two channels one for the therapeutic device, the other for suction.

The next set of injections may be given in the same area as the first or into the paravariceal tissues adjacent to the original ones. After each set of circumferential injections, withdraw the scope to slightly above the level that has been injected to begin the new set, stopping at the 30 cm level. Once the varices are obliterated in the distal esophagus, blood flow into the varices of the upper esophagus is impeded, causing these varices to diminish in size without direct treatment.

Although there is usually only a small amount of bleeding from each individual puncture site, slight oozing to rapid bleeding may occur. Occasionally, blood may be seen squirting from a varix after the needle has been removed. One to three further injections on either side of and/or below the bleeding site will usually stop persistent bleeding.

REMOVAL OF ENDOSCOPE

Following the last injection, the sclerotherapy needle should be removed from the accessory channel and discarded if disposable. The gastroscope is then advanced into the stomach. Suction is applied to decompress the gastric distention caused by continuous insufflation of air during the sclerotherapy treatment. The endoscope tip should remain in the stomach for approximately 5 min after completion of sclerotherapy. As it lies in the esophagus the endo-

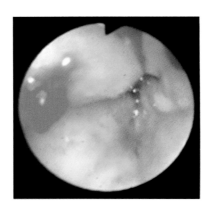

FIGURE 3.12 Immediately after treatment, multiple swollen mounds partially or completely obstruct the esophageal lumen. Since peristalsis is diminished acutely following EVS, decompression of the stomach should be performed by advancing the endoscope into the stomach to aspirate air.

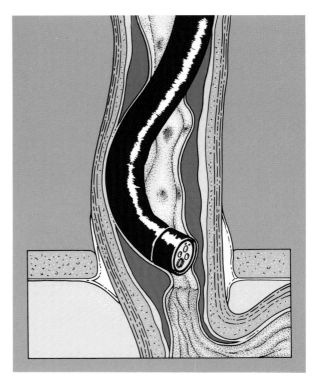

FIGURE 3.13 A bleeding puncture site may be tamponaded by torquing the flexed "knuckle" of the endoscope against the vessel. Note the swollen and "bruised" appearance of the injection sites.

scope tamponades, to some extent, the injection sites. Upon withdrawal, the esophagus may be completely dry or a small amount of oozing blood may be seen (Fig. 3.12). If free-flowing blood is encountered, suction will enable identification of the bleeding site which then can be effectively tamponaded by the tip of the gastroscope, applying direct pressure through torque or by advancing the shaft onto the bleeding area (Fig. 3.13). Usually, after 2 min of direct pressure, no further bleeding occurs. As the instrument is further withdrawn, blood frequently is encountered on the left wall at the level of approximately 27 to 30 cm from the incisor teeth. This does not signify acute bleeding but represents the pool of blood accumulated during EVS which the esophagus, traumatized by the multiple injections, cannot clear with peristalsis. In this case it is comforting to know that injections have not been made above 30 cm, so blood above that level is not a result of active bleeding.

EMERGENCY ESOPHAGEAL VARICEAL SCLEROTHERAPY

In emergency EVS the approximate site of bleeding can usually be identified and multiple injections given around and distal to that area. A double or large channel gastroscope will permit better suction capability than a standard single channel instrument. Endotracheal intubation may be desirable to prevent aspiration of blood and fluid.

FOLLOW-UP

The first repeat endoscopic sclerotherapy may be performed in 1 week. At that time, the esophagus may have a variety of appearances:

- The varices may look completely unchanged with no evidence of ulcer and no visible sites of puncture wounds.
- One or two discrete ulcerations may appear in the distal esophagus at the sites of previous injections (Figs. 3.14, 3.15).
- Marked ulcerations, friability, and diffuse erythema may be present (Fig. 3.16).

If the esophagus is free of ulcers, repeat the same technique described above. If ulcerations are present but not extensive, EVS may be performed avoiding the areas of obvious ulceration. No further attempt at EVS is indicated in the presence of extensive ulcerations.

Intervals between subsequent EVS sessions are at the discretion of the physician. The patient may be requested to return every 1 to 4 weeks for the remainder of the sessions, or to return monthly for several sessions, following which the intervals may be lengthened.

The recurring inflammation and cicatrization that follows EVS necrosis and healing of the wall usually result in perivariceal fibrosis, giving some protection

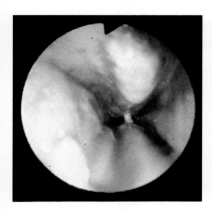 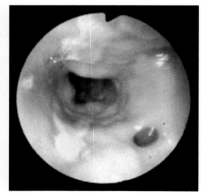 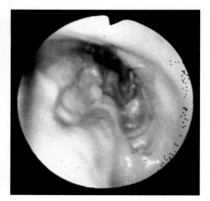

FIGURE 3.14 Superficial ulcerations are seen a few days after sclerotherapy.

FIGURE 3.15 Superficial ulcerations 1 week following sclerotherapy, along with a deeper ulceration which have the appearance of an esophageal diverticulum. All of these healed spontaneously within a month.

FIGURE 3.16 Deep discrete ulcerations 1 week following sclerotherapy. No treatment is given at this time and subsequent sclerotherapy is postponed for several weeks to permit healing.

against further bleeding episodes. However, until all varices are eradicated the patient is at risk for rebleeding. Complete eradication of varices may require several endoscopic sessions, or may occur early in the patient's course, with an average of 5 EVS sessions for complete disappearance of varices (Figs. 3.17, 3.18).

There is a recurrence of varices in 10 percent of patients once they are varix-free. Annual endoscopic checkups are recommended.

COMPLICATIONS

Complications of EVS occur in about 2% of patients and include esophageal ulceration (which may be confluent) (Figs. 3.19, 3.20), mediastinitis, pleural effusion, sepsis, confined perforation extending into the wall of the esophagus, bleeding, and stricture. Gastric varices have been known to develop. Mortality from this procedure is extremely rare and persis-

tent bleeding due to endoscopic injection of varices is distinctly unusual.

Variceal rebleeding may require repeat EVS or treatment with intravenous pressor agents. The Sengstaken-Blakemore balloon may induce excessive esophageal necrosis and should not be used if bleeding occurs in the immediate postinjection period. Transhepatic embolization may solve a recurrent bleeding problem temporarily, but failed EVS with persistent bleeding is an indication for surgical decompression.

Esophageal strictures are not unusual and the presence of a stricture usually indicates the disappearance of varices since the same fibrotic reparative process that causes dysphagia obliterates venous return. Even if the varices have not completely disappeared, the cicatricial reaction permits bougienage dilation without variceal bleeding. The strictures usually respond to one or two dilation sessions, and are rarely a cause of persistent symptoms (Fig. 3.21). Mucosal tags

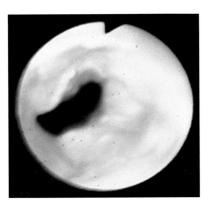

FIGURE 3.17 Complete absence of varices 4 months after sclerotherapy. Contrast this with the immediate post-procedure appearance seen in Figure 3.12.

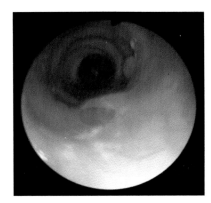

FIGURE 3.18 Follow-up 4 years after sclerotherapy completely obliterated esophageal varices. Note the re-epithelialized depressed scar from EVS. No recurrence could be identified.

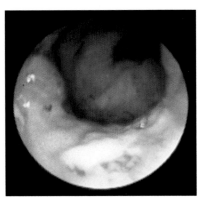

FIGURE 3.19 Chronic esophageal ulcers may occur secondary to EVS. This elderly patient's chronic ulcer may be due in part to persistent reflux through the hiatus hernia.

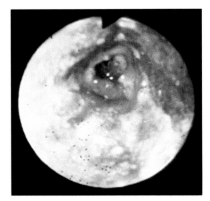

FIGURE 3.20 Diffuse superficial necrosis may follow EVS, as it did in this patient 1 week after the first sclerotherapy session.

(pseudopolyps) caused by ulceration and subsequent healing are commonly found following sclerotherapy, which may also lead to depressed scars and/or bridging (Figs. 3.22–3.25).

GASTRIC VARICES

Gastric varices do not respond as well to sclerotherapy as do those in the esophagus. Needle puncture of a gastric varix may be associated with prolonged bleeding from the injection site. This is difficult to tamponade and the bleeding may be problematic.

ESOPHAGEAL VARICEAL LIGATION (EVL)

An alternate method for eradication of esophageal varices has recently been described, esophageal variceal ligation (EVL). This technique utilizes a principle similar to that used in the rubberband ligation of hemorrhoids. A stretched rubberband is placed onto a cap which fits over the end of the gastroscope. Following identification of a varix, suction is applied through the endoscope suction channel, pulling a piece of mucosa along with the varix into the "well"

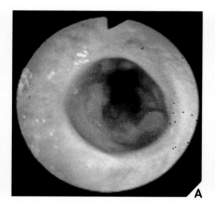 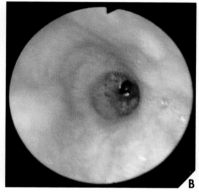 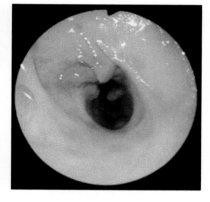

FIGURE 3.21 A circumferential stricture in the distal esophagus may result from sclerotherapy. When this happens, most of the varices are obliter-ated **(A)**. Follow-up 1 year later **(B)**. The stricture responded to bougie-nage dilations. Note the continued absence of esophageal varices.

FIGURE 3.22 Multiple pseudopolyps with a circumferential scar. Scars and pseudopolyps are common following eradication of varices.

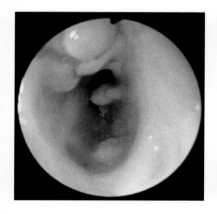 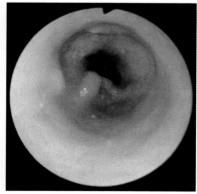 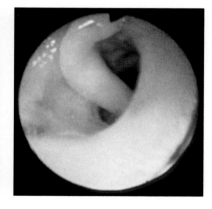

FIGURE 3.23 A narrowed lumen with pseudopolyps. The residual postin-flammatory pseudopolyps should not be confused with persistent varices.

FIGURE 3.24 Two adjacent pseu-dopolyps. Note their discrete charac-ter, which distinguishes them from varices which are usually longitudinal.

FIGURE 3.25 A re-epithelialized tube connected at both ends following sclerotherapy. This is a "bridge," sim-ilar to those seen in inflammatory bowel disease.

created by having affixed the cap onto the endoscope (Fig. 3.26).

Upon release of a trip-wire, the rubberband slides off the cap surrounding the base of the sucked-in piece of mucosa and varix, resulting in immediate strangulation with subsequent necrosis and fibrosis of that segment (refer to Fig. 3.26). The disposable rubberband-loaded cap must be replaced for ligation of additional varices. This is accomplished by removing the instrument from the esophagus and resetting another cap with its stretched rubberband. Multiple passes of the instrument are facilitated by back-loading an overtube onto the gastroscope prior to its initial insertion and sliding this into the upper esophagus where it remains during the course of examination.

The technique is rapid and relatively simple to use. Widespread experience is being accumulated in a method that appears to be a safe alternative to injection sclerotherapy in the treatment of both acute variceal bleeding and for the obliteration of esophageal varices.

REFERENCES

Sivak MV Jr, Blue MG: Endoscopic sclerotherapy of esophageal varices. In: Silvis SE, ed. *Therapeutic Gastrointestinal Endoscopy* 2nd ed. New York, NY: Igaku-Shoin; 1990:42.

Terblanche J, Krige JE, Bornman PC: Endoscopic sclerotherapy. *Surg Clin North Am* 1990;2:341.

Van Stiegmann G: Techniques for endoscopic obliteration of esophageal varices *Surg Ann* 1991;23:175.

Young HS, Matsui SM, Gregory PB: Sclerotherapy. In: Yamada T, ed. *Textbook of Gastroenterology* Philadelphia, Penn: JB Lippincott Co.; 1991:2601.

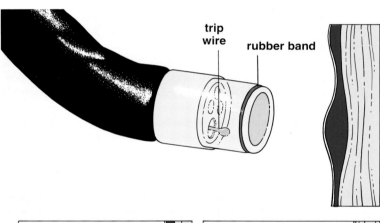

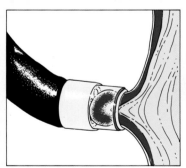
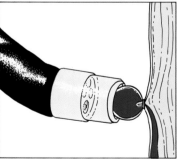

FIGURE 3.26 During esophageal variceal ligation, suction is applied through the endoscope suction channel. This pulls mucosa along with the varix into the cuff. Upon the release of the trip-wire, the rubberband slides off the cap resulting in immediate strangulation with subsequent necrosis and fibrosis of the segment.

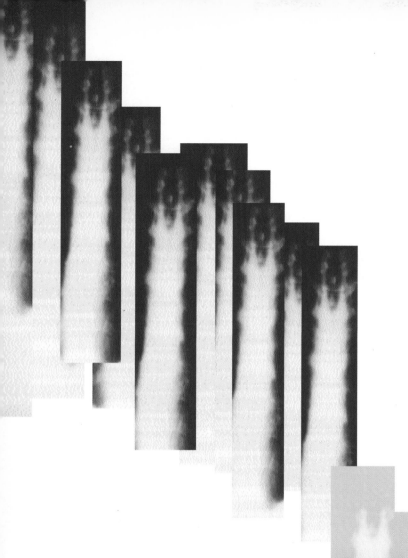

Treatment of Esophageal and Other Gastrointestinal Cancers

David Fleischer, MD

4

INTRODUCTION

Two factors have fostered the growth of endoscopic therapy for gastrointestinal (GI) cancers. First, many GI cancers do not cause symptoms until they are far advanced, at which time cure by surgical resection may not be possible. Second, the concept of minimally invasive surgery has continued to flourish. Although laporoscopic cholecystectomy focused the attention of general surgeons and the public on this concept, many current therapeutic endoscopic procedures are in fact surgical procedures performed via an endoscope. Endoscopic therapy for GI neoplasms is an important option for palliation in many patients with GI neoplasms. The focus of this chapter is the various endoscopic techniques available for therapy of esophageal cancer. The largest number of endoscopic options have been employed at this site and many of the principles for GI cancer treatment at other sites are similar. Some comment will be made on gastric and colorectal tumors. The endoscopic management of biliary and pancreatic cancers will be addressed in Chapters 8 and 9.

ESOPHAGEAL CANCER

For years the main role of the GI physician in the treatment of esophageal cancer was to determine whether or not the patient should be referred to the surgeon or the radiotherapist. Occasionally, he would dilate the tumor to provide temporary relief from dysphagia. The situation now is quite different. The palliative treatment options for the esophageal cancer patient (Tables 4.1, 4.2), indicate that not only may the endoscopist be involved with dilation, he also may be treating the cancer with a laser or some other thermal device, placing an endoscopic prosthesis, or inserting a gastrostomy tube. Various techniques will be described in this chapter, highlighting their advantages and disadvantages and attempting to place them in perspective. Primary esophageal tumors and proximal stomach carcinomas that grow beyond the esophagogastric junction into the esophagus will be considered together.

Symptoms of esophageal cancer may be caused by obstruction, bleeding, or a fistula. Several therapeutic modalities have been used to manage obstruction, but little information exists to allow one to determine which treatment is most appropriate or, if a combination of therapies is employed, what their sequence should be (Fig. 4.1). However, a few generalizations can be made.

In the unusual circumstance that the tumor is localized and there is no evidence of extension in an operative candidate, surgery is the treatment of choice. For tumors in the proximal half of the esophagus and for those that have spread, surgery is a poor choice for palliation because of high morbidity and mortality. Current imaging techniques

---

TABLE 4.1 PALLIATIVE TREATMENT OPTIONS FOR ESOPHAGEAL CANCER

- Surgery
- Radiotherapy
- Chemotherapy
- Endsocopic therapy
- Support only

TABLE 4.2 ENDOSCOPIC OPTIONS FOR PALLIATION OF ESOPHAGEAL CANCER

Thermal
- Laser ablation
- Photodynamic therapy
- After loading (intraluminal radiotherapy)
- Bipolar electrocoagulation (BICAP®)

Chemical
- Injection therapy

Mechanical
- Dilation
- Prosthesis
- Percutaneous endoscopic gastrostomy

underestimate the extent of the cancer and are not good predictors of resectability.

There is not a single prospective study comparing radiation therapy to surgery. Benefits from treatment with radiation therapy may not begin until 3 to 5 weeks after the onset of therapy. If a maximum dose is given–usually 5,000 to 6,000 rads–retreatment is not possible.

Only premature data on the benefits of chemotherapy exists. Some very encouraging results have been obtained using a regimen of cisplatin and fluorouracil. Chemotherapy is often used in conjunction with other therapies.

Dilation has been a useful adjunct to managing of malignant obstruction for years. Eventually, benefits are diminished and discomfort increased.

Endoscopic prostheses (stents) are extremely valuable for treatment of esophagorespiratory fistulae. They have also been used in patients with recurrent or progressive stenoses. A wider variety of shapes, designs, and delivery systems has increased their utility.

Although gastrostomy/jejunostomy offers an avenue by which nutrition can be poured into the digestive tract, it is not desirable for most patients as the only therapy because it deprives them of the pleasure of eating. Conceivably the gastrostomy site could provide a port of entry for an endoscopic procedure but usually this is technically difficult. In those patients who require a gastrostomy it can be performed as a percutaneous endoscopic procedure, if an endoscope can be advanced beyond the neoplastic obstruction and there are no contraindications (refer to Chapter 5).

For the rare esophageal tumor that is polypoid, endoscopic polypectomy is an effective way to remove neoplastic tissue. Endoscopic laser therapy (ELT) allows the physician to assess the tumor and to destroy part of the lesion under direct visualization by

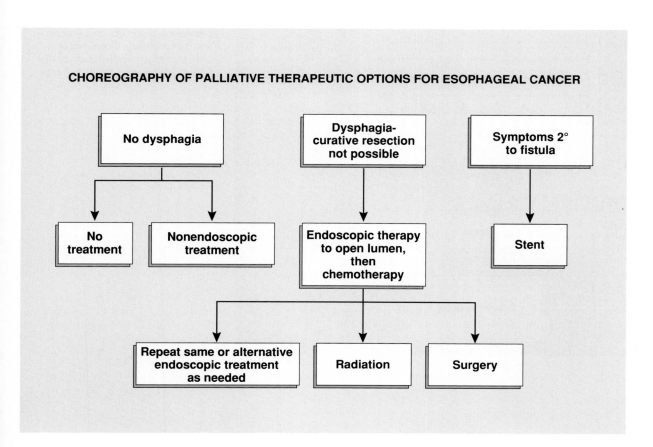

FIGURE 4.1 Algorithm showing the different palliative therapeutic options available for esophageal cancer.

thermal energy. Newly developed bipolar electrocoagulation probes have shown promise in a small group of patients.

ENDOSCOPIC LASER THERAPY

The word "laser" is an acronym for light amplification by stimulated emission of radiation. This phenomenon occurs when a substance is excited to a higher energy state and stimulated to emit light when it returns to its resting state. Because laser light is monochromatic it will have a predictable interaction with the tissue at which it is directed. Because it is coherent and collimated, it can be intensely and precisely aimed (Fig. 4.2).

Each type of laser has a discrete wavelength that determines its properties. To date, three types of lasers—argon, neodymium:yttrium aluminum garnet (Nd:YAG), and dye lasers—have been used for the endoscopic therapy of GI diseases. With the argon laser the active medium is a gas, while with the Nd:YAG it is solid. The dye laser utilizes organic dyes in liquid solutions and its principle, slightly distinct from the argon and YAG laser, will be discussed further in the section on photodynamic therapy. The distinctive features of each of these three lasers are listed in Table 4.3. Many types of lasers are used in other areas of medicine and surgery but have not

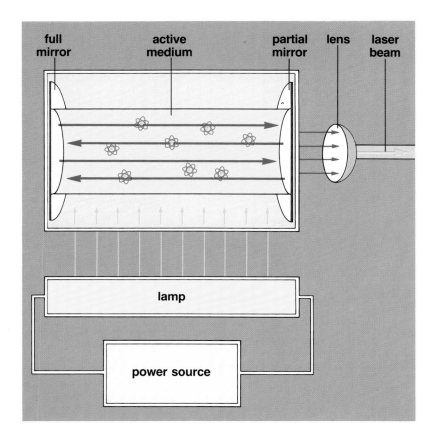

FIGURE 4.2 The principles of laser physics. A substance is excited to a higher energy state by a power source. In its efforts to reach a resting state, this substance gives off a photon of light. If it is placed between two mirrors, this process can be amplified. If one mirror is only partially reflective, part of the light will escape as the laser beam.

been employed for GI endoscopy, either because no specific application has as yet been identified or because they cannot be adapted for use with flexible endoscopes, usually because the proper waveguide does not exist.

The Nd:YAG is the most popular laser for GI neoplasms. As is the case with the Nd:YAG laser and from a practical point of view, the tissue event is determined by the temperature generated at the treatment site (Table 4.4). As a general guideline, protein coagulates at 60°C and tissue vaporizes at 100°C. The endoscopist estimates what is occurring by the tissue reaction. Coagulation creates a white blanched appearance with edema. With vaporization, a divot may occur, tissue often chars, and smoke may arise.

With any given laser, the endoscopist can control factors that influence the tissue event. More heating occurs with higher powers, longer pulse durations, and closer distances. Since heating is proportional to the cumulative thermal energy, tissue temperature rises more quickly if the pause between serial pulses is reduced.

INDICATIONS

Although the exact indication for endoscopic laser therapy (ELT) versus other treatment modalities is not

TABLE 4.3 TYPES OF MEDICAL LASERS IN COMMON USE

Type	Wavelength (μ)	Depth of penetration	Eye visibility	Medium
Nd:YAG	1.06	Least superficial	No	Solid
Argon	0.50	Intermediate	Yes	Gas
Dye	0.36-0.67	Most superficial	Yes	Liquid

TABLE 4.4 RELATIONSHIP BETWEEN TEMPERATURE AND TISSUE REACTION IN LASER THERAPY

Critical temperature	Histologic event	Endoscopic manifestation
45° C	Cell death, edema, endothelial damage, vasodilation	Erythema, edema cuff
60° C	Protein coagulates	Tissue turns white, blood turns black
80° C	Denatured collagen contracts, blood vessels constrict	Tissue "puckers"
100° C	Tissue water boils	Vaporization causes a divot
210° C +	Dehydrated tissue burns	Blackened tissue disappears or glowing embers appear

well defined, there are good and poor prognostic indices for the outcome of ELT (Fig. 4.3).

When the tumor is primarily mucosal (exophytic) it is easier to define borders between normal and abnormal tissue and easier to determine where to aim the laser beam. Submucosal (extrinsic) tumors are more difficult to treat because it is harder to define where the beam should be aimed and often impossible to keep the beam in the luminal axis. Additionally, if it is necessary to burn through normal tissue to destroy tumor, the treatment will be painful. Finally, restenosis is more likely to occur (Fig. 4.4).

The tumor's location also influences outcome. The outcome is best if the tumor is in a straight segment of the esophagus, particularly in the mid or distal portion. Tumors just beyond the cricopharyngeal juncture present unique problems. First, it is often difficult to position the endoscope if the tumor arises at or just beyond the sphincter. Damage to the endoscope is increased if there is little room to work. A separate problem is the disparity between technical

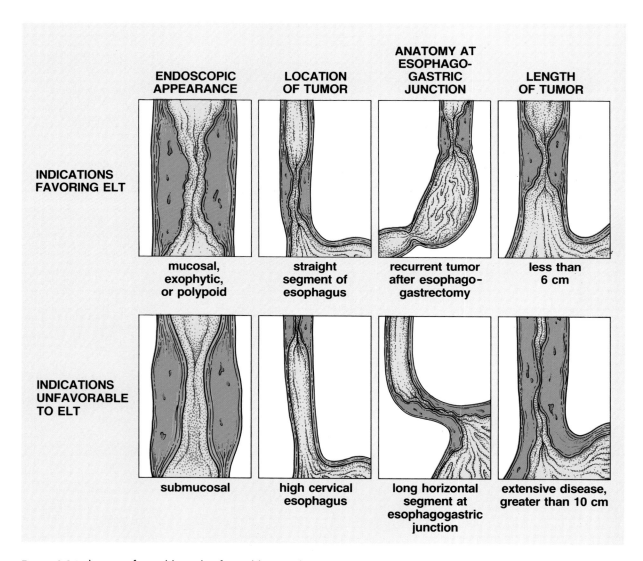

FIGURE 4.3 Indications favorable and unfavorable to endoscopic laser therapy for esophageal cancer.

TREATMENT OF ESOPHAGEAL AND OTHER GI CANCERS

success (opening the lumen) and functional success (ability to swallow effectively). Neuromuscular incoordination may cause dysphagia even in the face of a patent lumen.

If the tumor is in a long horizontal segment, as may be seen at the esophagogastric junction or after surgery, treatment is technically difficult and the patient's clinical response is poorer because drainage by gravity is impeded. Conversely, following esophagogastrectomy, the area of tumor recurrence is usually short and therefore more readily amenable to laser therapy.

The length of the tumor also has prognostic implications. Shorter tumors require fewer laser sessions. More extensive tumors take longer to debulk to achieve luminal opening and are usually at a more advanced stage so the patient's downhill course is more rapid.

Initial Assessment

Initial consideration for endoscopic laser therapy (ELT) for palliative treatment must answer these questions:

- Is the patient a candidate?
- What are the goals of treatment?
- Is ancillary therapy planned?

In determining the patient's candidacy, the physician must assure himself and the patient that curative surgery is not possible. Usually an imaging study of the chest and abdomen demonstrates whether curative therapy is an option. Findings which vote against cure are listed in Table 4.5. If there is any possibility for cure and there are no medical contraindications, exploratory surgery should be performed. The patient is also not a candidate for ELT if his functional status is so poor that even if the lumen were opened, it would not greatly alter his quality of life. Both the physician and the patient must be clear on the goals of laser therapy. The patient must understand that it is a palliative measure and that it will be temporary. The physician must define his endpoint prior to therapy, which is usually relief of obstruction quickly and safely. If ancillary treatment is to follow–for example, radiation therapy–the goal may be to open the lumen

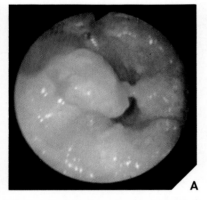

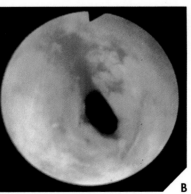

Figure 4.4 Esophageal cancer. Exophytic—predominantly mucosal—tumors **(A)** are readily amenable to ELT since a shelf of tumor tissue is generally accessible. Submucosal tumors **(B)** are more difficult to treat because there is no distinct ledge at which to aim the laser beam.

TABLE 4.5 FINDINGS THAT SUGGEST A CURATIVE THERAPY IS UNLIKELY FOR ESOPHAGEAL CANCER

- Radiographic length > 5 cm
- Deviation and angulation of the esophageal axis
- Obliteration of peri-esophageal fat planes
- Invasion of trachea or bronchi
- Invasion of aorta
- Liver or bone metastasis

only enough to relieve dysphagia. If all other therapies have been exhausted, more extensive treatment may be the goal. Relief of dysphagia is a realistic goal. Relief of pain is not. An important question is how ELT fits into the scheme of combined therapy but, unfortunately, little is known about the benefits or risks of combination therapy, proper sequence, or timing. For this reason, the patient's first visit should include evaluation by a team of physicians, including a surgeon, oncologist, radiation therapist, and GI endoscopist.

PATIENT EVALUATION

In addition to a complete blood count and biochemical tests (multichemical analyses), three examinations are required to assess suitability for laser therapy and to plan treatment. They are a barium swallow, an endoscopy, and an imaging study of the chest and abdomen. All these tests have prognostic implications. The barium swallow defines the location and extent of the tumor. This will affect technical decisions and help assess the number of treatments required. The endoscopy allows the physician to see the gross appearance of the tumor, and obtain biopsies and cytologies to establish or confirm the diagnosis of cancer.

Until recently, the imaging study was almost always a CT scan. Endoscopic ultrasonography (EUS) is a new technology which may give complementary or, at times, more precise information. With EUS, the ultrasound crystal can be placed into the tip of the endoscope. Since the probe enters the lumen, there is an opportunity to obtain information about both the depth of tumor penetration and local lymph node involvement. The imaging study serves to define the extent of the disease. The CT scan often underestimates the extent and cannot be used as the sole guide for resectability. With radiographic imaging, biopsies may often be obtained to establish the nonresectability of the tumor. In addition, the imaging study may be valuable in planning the therapy's technical details. Figure 4.5 shows the barium swallow of a patient who developed recurrent adenocarcinoma at the anastomosis in the chest following resection for cancer of the gastric cardia. The CT scan precisely defines the anatomy outside the lumen, showing the endoscopist that at the narrowed anastomotic site the wall is thick enough to allow him to attempt ELT. Had the diameter of the wall been thin like the normal esophageal wall, ELT would have been ruled out because of the high likelihood of perforation.

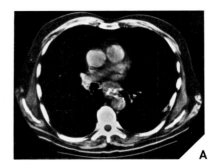

A

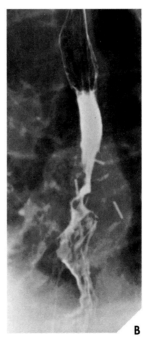

B

FIGURE 4.5 Combined use of barium swallow and CT scan of chest to plan laser therapy. The CT scan precisely defines the anatomy surrounding the structure (**A**). The barium swallow doesn't clearly show what the thickness of the tissue surrounding the stricture in this patient with recurrent adenocarcinoma after esophagogastrectomy (**B**).

PATIENT PREPARATION

In the United States, ELT for esophageal cancer usually begins as an inpatient procedure. It is possible that follow-up examinations, often including additional laser therapy, can be done as an outpatient procedure. The treatment is performed where the laser is housed. Patients are usually sedated with meperidine and midazolam intravenously. If the lumen is completely obstructed or the tumor is high in the cervical esophagus an anticholinergic drug is added to decrease secretions. General anesthesia is seldom required. In the procedure room, the equipment is shown to the patient and he is apprised of what he may feel, hear, and smell. The procedure is done in the standard left lateral decubitus endoscopic position. Generally two more health personnel—other physicians and/or nurses or GI assistants—help during the procedure, one attending the patient and the equipment, the other circulating and recording medical observations. The most recent barium swallow is displayed on the view box.

ENDOSCOPIC LASER THERAPY
SURVEILLANCE ENDOSCOPY

The procedure begins with a surveillance endoscopy with a small diameter endoscope. If possible, the entire tumor is viewed endoscopically to assess the geography of the lesion.

- What is the actual length of the tumor?
- How much is exophytic and how much is submucosal?
- Where are the points of obstruction? It is important to note where these ledges of obstruction occur.

The location of the biopsy port will vary with different instruments—usually it is between 4 o'clock and 8 o'clock. This will affect the ease or difficulty with which lesions on a specific side—left or right—will be aligned for treatment. One wants to know if there are sharp turns and if a bigger double channel endoscope can pass through the tumor. The double channel scope has two important advantages:

- One channel can be used for smoke and gas exhaust while the other is used for the fiber.
- Because there are two biopsy ports, the fiber can exit at either 4 o'clock or 7 o'clock, depending upon which channel is used for the laser fiber and which for the gas exhaust. This versatility is often of great benefit when aiming the beam at a ledge in a particular direction. Often the larger scope cannot be used until after the lumen is dilated.

As videoendoscopy has become more popular, there are specific advantages to using it for laser therapy. It is not necessary to wear protective eyeglasses and the exhaust fumes are not likely to be inhaled. However, at the present time, a wide variety of instruments—smaller size, double channel—are not readily available.

TECHNIQUE

After completing the surveillance endoscopy, one usually finds that only a small, single channel endoscope passes through the tumor and frequently not even that. When ELT was initially developed for esophageal cancer, treatment began at the upper level of the tumor. Although this approach is less favored now, it still has considerable merit. Today it is more common to dilate the tumor so that one can get an endoscope to the distal margin and have the option of beginning therapy at the inferior portion of the tumor.

This is accomplished by passing small diameter endoscope through the tumor to the antrum. A 1.8 mm guidewire with scored markings is passed through its biopsy channel. The markings on the wire are scored at preselected distances from the tip, such as two marks at 40 cm, three marks at 60 cm, etc. There are seven markings, and by multiplying the number of markings by 20 the distance in cm from the tip can be calculated. The endoscopist should leave the distal tip of the wire in the midantrum which is approximately 60 cm from the incisors. The endoscope is then removed, keeping the guidewire in place. This is accomplished by advancing the guidewire 10 cm and then withdrawing the endoscope 10 cm. By using measurements obtained previously, the distance from the midantrum to the incisors is known. The guidewire markings close to this juncture are now the key landmarks to its proper positioning. In most cases, with the tip of the guidewire in the midantrum, three marks, denoting 60 cm, are seen at the incisors (Fig. 4.6).

Progressively larger polyvinyl tapered dilators are passed over the guidewire. The dilators also have measured markings so one can better assess where resistance from the tumor mass is met. Hopefully the lumen can be enlarged to allow for the passage of a double channel 13 mm endoscope, but this is seldom possible. Nonetheless, dilation is usually effective enough to allow treatment to begin at the distal tumor margin (Fig. 4.7).

If not even the smallest endoscope will pass beyond the obstruction, the endoscopist has two options. He may begin treatment at the proximal margin or he may dilate the tumor. If he chooses the latter approach, fluoroscopic assistance will be required unless he knows from the barium swallow or from previous examination that there is straight passage.

After the guidewire is passed, dilation is carried out as described above.

What are the advantages and disadvantage of beginning the treatment distally? The overall goal of ELT for esophageal cancer is to remove the luminal obstruction and relieve symptoms of dysphagia. This is more desirable if it can be accomplished safely in a short period. If treatment begins at the proximal margin, the edema that forms with the laser burn usually reduces the luminal size initially. Therefore, after the proximal margin is burned, it is difficult to get the scope more distally to treat the tumor at other levels. However, if the treatment starts at the most distal point, as the endoscope is withdrawn proximally for continued treatment, the edema that is formed is not a problem (Fig. 4.8). The primary appeal of starting ELT distally is that the endoscopist can treat the entire length of the tumor in a single session, potentially diminishing the total number of laser sessions required to open the lumen.

Naturally there are trade-offs. The treatment of the proximal margin is usually the easiest technically because the view is *en face*. The beam is easily focused

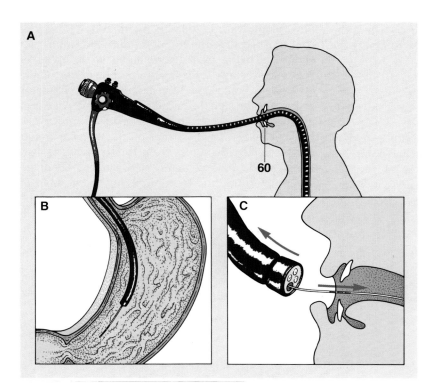

FIGURE 4.6 A small diameter endoscope is passed beyond the tumor into the antrum. The endoscopist notes the markings on the endoscope at the incisors (eg, 60 cm) when the tip is in the midantrum (**A**). A flexible guidewire is passed through the biopsy port (**B**). Alternatively, the endoscope is withdrawn approximately 10 cm and then the guidewire is "pushed out" about 10 cm. This allows the endoscope to be withdrawn but the guidewire to be left in the stomach at approximately 60 cm. The position is confirmed by noting the scored markings on the guidewire. The number of markings times 20 equals the distance in cm from the tip of the guidewire. If the endoscopist desires the guidewire to be in the midantrum (eg, 60 cm), the three markings should be positioned at the incisors (**C**).

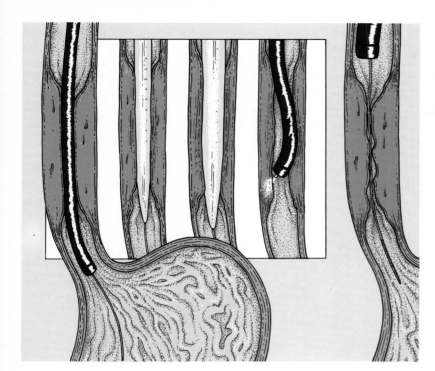

FIGURE 4.7 After the guidewire has been placed through the endoscope, progressively larger dilators can be passed. After dilation, it will be possible to begin treatment at the distal tumor margin. If the endoscope will not pass the obstruction and it is known that the tumor is in a straight segment of the esophagus, guidewire passage can be carried out and dilation performed.

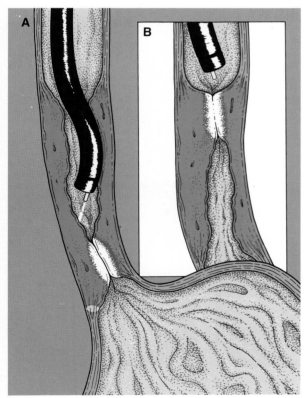

FIGURE 4.8 Immediate effect of laser burn is thermal damage and tissue swelling which may narrow the lumen. When laser therapy is begun distally, the edema will not impede treatment since the scope will be pulled cephalad (**A**). When treatment is begun at the proximal margin, edema will prevent advancement of the scope in a caudad direction and therefore therapy will be limited to only one area (**B**). New edema in treated areas noted in white.

close to the lumen. The burn proceeds in concentric circles, moving toward but not onto the normal esophageal wall (Fig. 4.9). The tumor tissue is pinkish red. After initial coagulative damage it becomes white. Further heating vaporizes the tissue, turning it black and creating divots (Figs. 4.10- 4.12).

If the lumen is not severely narrowed, it may be possible to begin ELT distally and get a relatively good *en face* view. However, often the luminal narrowing is severe and treatment begun distally requires use of a small endoscope and a tangential approach with the endoscope and the fiber in awkward positions (Fig. 4.13). This enhances the risk of perforation because the laser beam is no longer fired directly along the axis of the lumen and the endoscope's tip is extremely close to the treatment site. This is also problematic because carbon debris deposits on the distal lens obscure the view, and because the risk of damage to the endoscope is increased. The other concern with distal treatment is overdistention. With the endoscope jammed into the lumen it is difficult for gas to escape proximally.

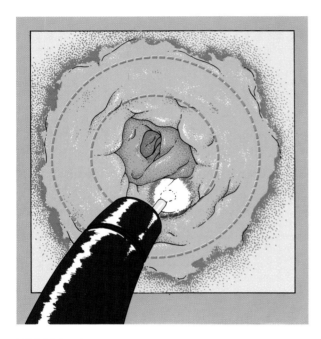

FIGURE 4.9 When endoscopic laser therapy must be delivered to the proximal margin of the tumor, the best approach is *en face*. The endoscope is positioned above the proximal tumor margin with the laser beam perpendicular to the tumor surface. The initial burn will be delivered centrally and circumferentially around the lumen. Further burns will be delivered in concentric circles toward, but not onto the normal esophageal wall.

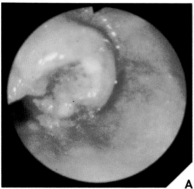
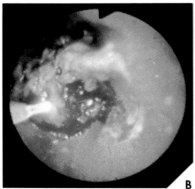
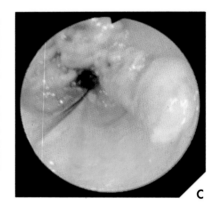

A   B   C

FIGURE 4.10 Esophageal tumor treated by endoscopic laser therapy. Bulky mucosal esophageal cancer. Exophytic type of tumor lends itself to treatment (**A**). Laser fiber delivering treatment seen at 8 o'clock . White coagulum noted at superior margin. Some self-limited bleeding, is seen (**B**). After laser therapy tumor, bulk is reduced. White coagulum is seen (**C**).

Some is suctioned into the lumen but the majority passes distally. The endoscopist must palpate the abdomen periodically and check with the patient and nurses frequently to determine the degree of distention.

There is general consensus but not unanimity regarding laser settings. Most commonly the tumor is destroyed by vaporization, which is generally achieved with settings of 80 to 100 W for 2 sec or greater at distances of approximately 1 cm. Because of beam divergence, the laser tip should be close to the tumor. The 1 cm distance is an estimate. A small number of laser endoscopists prefer to use lower energies in the range of 50 W to accomplish tumor destruction by coagulation because, although this is a slower process, less smoke is generated. The plume of smoke containing gas, cells, and carbon debris is the major technical limitation to vaporization. Deposits of

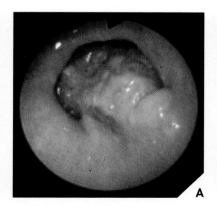

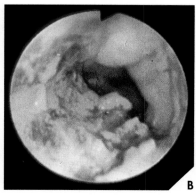

FIGURE 4.11 Exophytic esophageal cancer seen prior to laser therapy. Lesion is ideal for laser therapy as protruding exophytic portion is readily treated (**A**). Two days postprocedure. White necrotic tumor could readily be debrided. Dilation is effective for removing loose necrotic tissue (**B**).

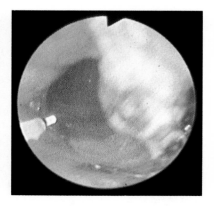

FIGURE 4.12 Esophageal tumor. With further treatment, vaporization and divoting occur. Smoke is given off.

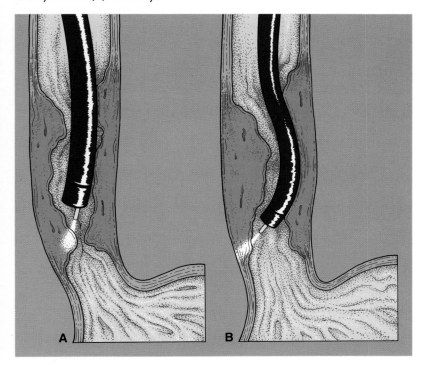

FIGURE 4.13 Endoscope in lumen delivering laser therapy to distal tumor ledge. *En face* approach possible because luminal narrowing is not severe (**A**). Lumen is so constricted that in order for the laser to be aimed at the distal tumor ledge, it must be bent at a very acute angle, meaning it is no longer parallel to the luminal axis, increasing the risk of perforation (**B**).

this material on the distal lens of the endoscope restrict vision. Unless the smoke can be successfully vented away, the endoscope will have to be removed intermittently for cleaning.

The treatment session for one day is normally completed when the maximal amount of tumor has been treated. At the end of the treatment the tissue is often charred black and edematous secondary to thermal damage. There may be some oozing from the friable neoplastic tissue but major blood loss is not a problem (Fig. 4.14).

POSTPROCEDURE

After the treatment the patient is kept NPO except for ice chips for 4 hrs. Swallowing is often worse after ELT due to edema which narrows the lumen. The patient, his family, the nurses, and other physicians involved in his care are apprised of this in advance to minimize concern. If the patient is stable the diet is advanced to clear liquids later that day. When the procedure was first performed, all patients were started on parenteral nutrition during the 4 or 5 laser sessions which extended over 10 days or longer. Now it is uncommon to require more than 3 sessions for any patient so parenteral nutrition is seldom instituted. Vital signs are checked hourly at first and then routinely. The patient may have some chest pain after the treatment. If there is odynophagia, antacids may relieve symptoms by coating the raw tumor surface. However, often there is chest pain because tumor tissue has been burned. Narcotic analgesics may be necessary. For the beginning laser therapist, it is wise to obtain chest x-ray and/or abdominal films to exclude a perforation. As one becomes more experienced, it is not necessary to order them routinely. It is common for there to be a low-grade fever and mild elevation in the white blood count 12 to 36 hrs after laser therapy.

Patients are routinely treated every other day until maximal luminal opening is achieved. This schedule

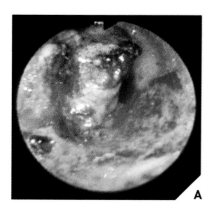

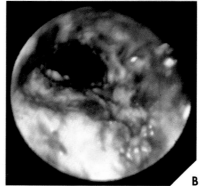

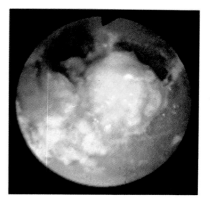

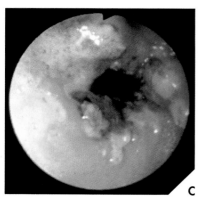

FIGURE 4.14 Appearance of cancer after endoscopic laser therapy session. Polypoid tumor in middle of esophageal lumen has a blackened, charred appearance (A). Several sites along course of esophageal cancer are black and charred after treatment (B). White coagulation changes at superior margin of tumor postprocedure (C).

FIGURE 4.15 Necrotic tumor tissue viewed 48 hrs after endoscopic laser therapy. It is yellow-white and of pudding-like consistency.

TREATMENT OF ESOPHAGEAL AND OTHER GI CANCERS

has several purposes. Maximal tumor necrosis will have occurred and debridement is facilitated. Patients often appreciate a "day off". Oral intake can be advanced in the interim. This also is beneficial to the physician's scheduling.

SUBSEQUENT SESSIONS

The second endoscopic procedure, 48 hrs after the first, begins with a surveillance endoscopy. The effects of the last treatment are noted. Usually the tissue that had been treated with the laser 2 days before is a yellow-white mass of pudding-like consistency (Fig. 4.15). The endoscope can be used to push this necrotic tissue distally into the stomach, in effect, using it to debride and dilate the tumor as well as to observe changes. During the endoscopy one decides whether further dilation is required before the next treatment, what endoscope and fiber will be used, and how much more laser treatment is necessary. Numerous accessories are available to remove necrotic tissue clogging the lumen (Fig. 4.16). If repeated intubations will be required to remove "chunks" of treated tissue, then an overtube can be used.

Dilators are commonly used because, like the endoscope, they can both debride and dilate. The

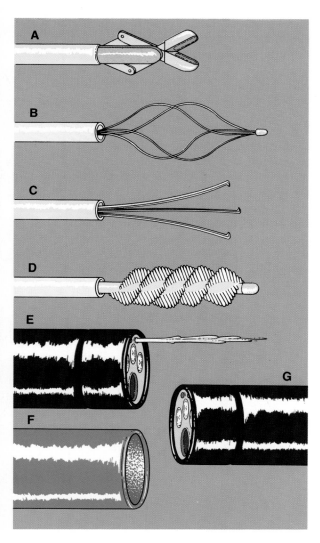

FIGURE 4.16 The dilator is the simplest to use to remove pudding-like debris, and also serves to enlarge the lumen. Other useful devices for debris removal:
- Biopsy forceps (**A**).
- Sphincterotomy basket (**B**).
- Polyp grasper (**C**).
- Endoscopic brush (**D**).
- Water jet (**E**).
- Large caliber suction tube—modified (**F**).
- Endoscope, used as a pusher (**G**).

endoscope is advanced into the stomach, the guidewire is passed, the endoscope removed, and the dilation begun. After the dilation, consideration is given to further therapy.

There is no fixed definition for the endpoint of therapy. It will depend in part on what ancillary treatment is planned and what the clinical situation dictates. However, it would be uncommon to halt ELT until at least an 11 mm, and usually a 13 mm endoscope could be passed.

Follow-Up

After the final endoscopic laser therapy, a barium swallow is obtained to make sure that no perforation has occurred and to document the effects of therapy (Fig. 4.17). Dietary recommendations can be made based on the degree of luminal opening and the patient's appetite and desires. Often, a liquid nutritional supplement, such as a milkshake with a raw egg mixed in, is advised. The importance of chewing foods well, avoiding stringy foods, and following solid foods with a liquid flush are stressed. Since there may be problems with appetite as well as mechanical obstruction which interfere with food intake, some tips about food preparation are give, to the person who will be preparing meals (Table 4.6). Medications are not routinely prescribed unless there is odynphagia for which antacids may be helpful.

The first follow-up endoscopy is usually carried out in 3 to 4 weeks unless the clinical situation dictates an earlier examination. A white exudate ordinarily coats the laser-treated area (Fig. 4.18). If minimal symptoms of dysphagia are present, a dilation may be done. If there is a regrowth of tumor and obstruction appears imminent, outpatient ELT is performed.

Related Complications

The incidence of perforation after ELT for esophageal cancer is 5% to 8%. Other complications include gaseous distention in 5% to 15% of patients. Goals of therapy are not achieved in 10% to 12% of patients. Damage to fibers and endoscopes is more common than during treatment of GI bleeding.

Safety Precautions for Health Personnel

There are some health concerns which endoscopy personnel using lasers need to consider. The light from the laser beam can cause retinal injury. With fiberoptic endoscopes, anyone who observes the treatment being performed should wear safety glasses. When endoscopic laser therapy (ELT) is performed with videoendoscopes, there is no need to wear protective glasses since the procedure is observed on a television monitor. Another safety advantage of videoendoscopy is that the control section of the endoscope does not need to be held to the physician's eye. Therefore, the smoke emitted from the endoscopic channels will not exit near the endoscopist's nose where it could be inhaled. There is still controversy as to whether the plume of smoke that is produced when tumor is vaporized contains dangerous elements. There is no information

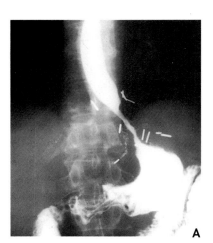 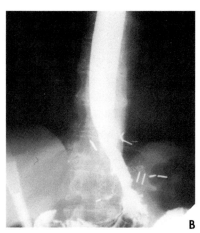

Figure 4.17 Barium swallow of carcinoma of the esophagogastric junction recurrent after surgery (**A**). The posttherapy radiograph shows increased luminal diameter and no evidence of perforation (**B**).

suggesting that viable tumor cells are in the plume, but some viral particles have been identified. Since their long term effect is unknown, it is wise to take appropriate precautions.

Health personnel should wear masks specifically designed to provide maximum protection against smoke inhalation. Routine surgical masks do not filter out the smallest particles. An endoscopy assistant should suction smoke from the patient's mouth to prevent it from spreading. The room should have good ventilation and exhaust fans. Skin burns are uncommon, but a policy should mandate that the laser must be in "standby" rather than "operate" mode when the fiber is not in the endoscope. A few cases of in the operating room fires have been reported. They have been associated with bronchoscopy, where oxygen was used, and in association with endotracheal tubes that ignited. Special care should be taken in the latter setting and specifically designed endotracheal tubes are available. During laparotomy, fires have

TABLE 4.6 TIPS FOR PREPARING MEALS FOR PATIENTS WITH ESOPHAGEAL CANCER

General
- Eat smaller meals more often. For example, one meal can be a small milkshake. Before and after each bite of food, drink nutritional supplement.
- Chew food slowly.
- Make sure all the liquids you drink have a nutritional content, such as milkshake, fruit juices, or supplements.
- Cut meats up into small bites and add gravy to them.
- Avoid acidic, salty, or highly spiced foods.
- Stay away from foods that were bothersome before laser treatments— if certain foods caused indigestion or bloating, avoid them.
- As soon as one feels "comfortably" full, stop eating.
- Avoid fried foods. Use methods such as baking, boiling, and pressure cooking. Try to make foods as moist as possible—use gravies, sauces, broth, etc. to moisten food whenever possible.
- Have the deli slice some meats very thin—ham, turkey, chicken.

Foods To Avoid
- Acidic, salty, or highly spiced foods. Clam chowder is sometimes difficult to get down.
- Rice in soups is often hard to swallow—too small.
- Stay away from fibrous meat, fish, or vegetables—lobster, scallops, bacon, chuck roast, hot dogs, steak, sausage, stems of broccoli, celery, certain forms of squash, asparagus, sweet potatoes, bean sprouts, peas, mushrooms, salads. On the other hand, steamed or raw oysters or clams are very easy to swallow.
- Cut away bread crust or the hard edge of macaroni or pastas. Spaghetti is sometimes difficult to swallow, whereas macaroni with a thinned sauce is very easy to swallow.
- Avoid the yolk of hard-boiled egg or dry, large curd cottage cheese.
- Avoid pure forms of chocolate—chocolate sauce, candy, or pudding—as well as peppermint.
- Stay away from high-fiber breads, cereals, nuts, and crackers.

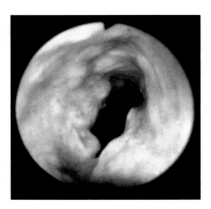

FIGURE 4.18 Typical white coating on wall of esophagus in areas treated by laser.

There are two accepted techniques for using the tumor probe—the antegrade and the retrograde. With the retrograde approach, the tumor probe is advanced beyond the distal tumor margin with fluoroscopic observations (refer to Fig. 4.22). Measurements on the shaft of the probe, the radiopaque markers, and the resistance as the probe traverses the tumor assist the endoscopist in properly locating the probe. Under fluoroscopy, the probe is then pulled retrograde, delivering a burn at several stations along the way, the

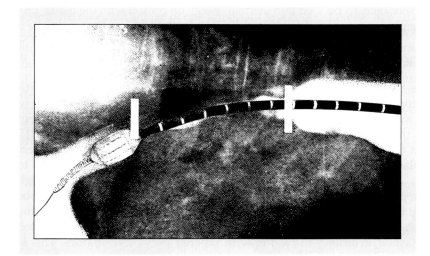

FIGURE **4.22** The tumor probe is passed over guidewire, through mouth, into and beyond distal tumor margin. Fluoroscopic picture showing markings on the probe shaft and radiopaque markers on patient's torso will help assure proper placement.

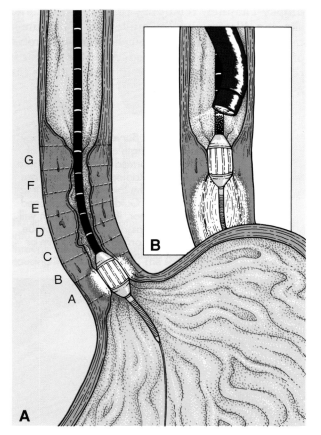

FIGURE **4.23** The probe is pulled retrograde until it engages the tumor. Endoscopist usually feels resistance at this point. Treatment is delivered at stations "A-G" along vertical axis of tumor, each station corresponding to the length of electrically active probe coils. The zone of injury extends 1 to 2 mm around lumen (**A**). A small caliber endoscope can be passed through the mouth alongside the shaft of the probe to assure that last burn is delivered precisely at proximal margin of tumor (**B**).

number of which is determined by the length of the tumor (refer to Fig. 4.23).

With the antegrade approach, the procedure begins in the same fashion. However, at the time that the tumor probe is passed over the guidewire and through the mouth, it is only advanced to the proximal margin of the tumor. At that point, a small caliber endoscope is also passed through the cricopharyngeus and into the upper esophagus. The tumor probe can then be viewed directly as it is advanced into the tumor. With this technique, the first burn is delivered at A (Fig. 4.24) and is observed directly. The endoscopist will hear the sound of the tissue burning and see smoke. The treated tissue will turn white or dark if it is hemorrhagic. If a probe is used with an activated treatment section of 1.5 cm, the probe is advanced through stations of 1 cm in length by observing the markers on the the tumor probe shaft descend into the tumor. The advance is also monitored fluoroscopically. By advancing at 1 cm intervals with a 1.5 cm active electrode, the endoscopist accepts a bit of overlap tissue heating.

This compensates for the fact that the procedure is not observed directly once the probe descends into the tumor, with hopes that the overlap may compensate for any imprecision in positioning. The treatment is complete when:

- The probe has passed through the number of 1 cm stations that correspond to the length of the area to be treated.
- The probe fluoroscopically passes beyond the distal marker on the patient's skin.
- A "give" is felt as the probe passes beyond the distal tumor margin.

Powers of 50 W are generally used and the probe is left at each station for 15 sec. Different treatment durations are required for different sized probes. These settings are available from the manufacturer.

The probe is removed and, if possible, the endoscope is passed through the lumen to observe the effects of thermal injury. If the injury has been perfectly delivered, a circumferential white burn is

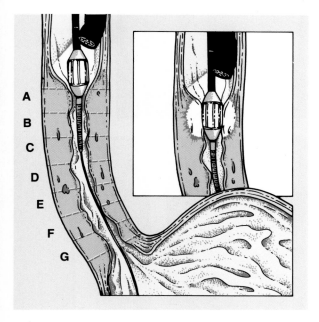

FIGURE 4.24 The antegrade approach. First burn is delivered at the point "A".

seen (Fig. 4.25). When it is incomplete, or if the probe pulls tissue with it as it advances, some areas will appear white while other areas will be friable and hemorrhagic (Fig. 4.26).

ENDOSCOPIC PROSTHESES

A variety of esophageal prostheses are available, the most common of which are made of latex or silicone rubber, polyvinyl chloride, or other plastic materials (Fig. 4.27). Expandable metal stents, similar to those used in the biliary tree, are being developed for application in the esophagus. The several methods of endoscopy-assisted insertion are variations on a single theme. They involve widening the lumen, usually by dilation, occasionally by thermal destruction of tumor, in preparation for insertion of the stent. The stent is forced into proper position and held there by the snug fit, anchoring flanges, and the adherence of the tumor to the prosthesis. There is universal agreement that this represents the best treatment for esophagorespiratory fistulae which may occur spontaneously or as a complication of endoscopic therapy (Fig. 4.28). There is little agreement as to what role stents have in managing of esophageal cancers not complicated by fistulae.

Various methods for placing stents have been well-chronicled and are referenced. The technique which this author finds easiest, safest, and most effective is described in detail below.

MEASUREMENT OF TUMOR
Using a small caliber endoscope, the proximal and distal margins of the tumor are precisely identified.

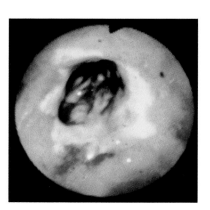

FIGURE 4.25 Circumferential white burn following tumor therapy by bipolar electro-coagulation.

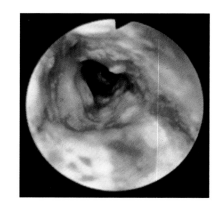

FIGURE 4.26 Typical tissue changes after electrocoagulation. Some areas show white burn. Other areas are friable and hemorrhagic.

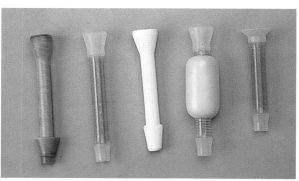

FIGURE 4.27 A variety of esophageal prostheses are commercially available. From left to right:
• Celestin-type (Bard)
• Normal flange (Wilson-Cook)
• Atkinson-Nottingham (Key-Med)
• Expandable (Wilson-Cook)
• Low profile, upper flange (Wilson-Cook)

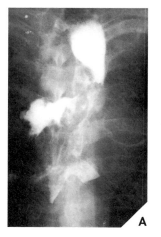
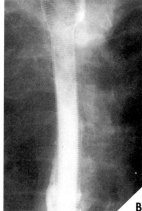

FIGURE 4.28 Esophageal cancer complicated by perforation. Note tracheoesophageal fistula (**A**). After placement of esophageal prosthesis, fistula is closed off and patient can ingest food orally (**B**).

The length of the tumor and the distance of each landmark from the incisors is of great importance in selecting the appropriate stent. Since most stents have a proximal flange 3 to 4 cm in length, it is also important to measure the location of the upper esophageal sphincter and its distance from the proximal tumor margin. If there is an esophagorespiratory fistula that is not within the narrowed tumor segment—proximal to it—it should be determined if the stent flange will cover it.

DILATION OF LUMEN

Most prostheses have outside diameters of 14 to 16mm. It is therefore necessary to dilate the lumen with firm dilators of at least 15 mm, although a 16 mm tapered polyvinyl dilator is preferable. Just what size the last dilator will be prior to stent placement requires some judgment. If the tumor is rigid and/or the mediastinum is fixed, use a dilator at least one size larger than the stent's outside diameter. For these tumors, it is safest not to stretch the lumen in a single

dilating session because the risk of perforation increases. One or more dilations, in addition to the one on the day of the stent, are usually carried out. On the other hand, if the tumor is either soft (as necrotic tumors may be) or rubbery, the last dilator should be the same diameter as the stent since they are more prone to migrate if the lumen is over-dilated. The stent can usually be inserted in these tumors on the day the initial dilation takes place.

EQUIPMENT

Commercial prostheses are now available in a wide variety of diameters and lengths. Other equipment required at the time of stent placement includes polyvinyl dilators, a guidewire, a modified longer dilator to be used as a stabilizer, a pusher tube, 3-0 silk suture at least 120 cm in length or fishing line of equivalent strength, silicone lubricant, an indelible marker, and an accessory to assist with stent removal if that is necessary.

STENT PLACEMENT

The procedure is performed using fluoroscopy. The exact location of the proximal and distal tumor margins (eg, such as 25 cm and 32 cm) from the incisors is confirmed for the final time. Some endoscopists confirm these spots with external radiopaque markers, but most find these inexact. Dilation is carried out over a guidewire placed in the proximal antrum and confirmed fluoroscopically.

In preparation for the actual stent placement, certain pieces of equipment have been readied. The 3-0 silk thread has been passed through a puncture site in the upper part of the flange. Its sole purpose is to aid in removing a poorly positioned stent. The thread is fed retrograde through the inside of the pusher tube and will be in position inside the pusher tube, exiting through its proximal end. The inside of the stent and pusher tube are lubricated with silicone prior to putting both of them over the stabilizing dilator (Fig. 4.29).

The pusher tube has been marked so that key points will be recognized during the passage of the stent and pusher. Choose a stent that has a shaft 3 cm longer than the tumor with a proximal flange that adds an additional 3 cm. For a 7 cm tumor, a stent 13 cm long would be used. If you plan for the top of the flange to sit at 22 cm, allow for 3 cm above the proximal margin of the tumor, and for the shaft to extend 3 cm beyond the distal tumor margin to 35 cm.

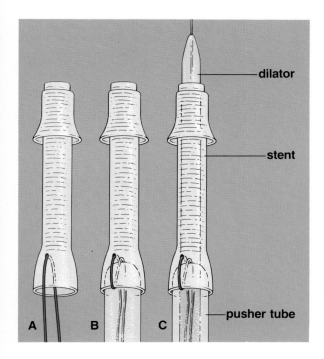

FIGURE 4.29 Through a puncture site made in the flange of the stent with a scalpel blade, the 3-0 silk suture is fed (**A**). The suture is fed retrograde inside the lumen of the pusher tube (**B**). Stent and pusher tube placed over stabilizing dilator (**C**). Note suture is inside pusher lumen, exiting at proximal end.

The pusher tube is marked anew using an indelible pen for each stent to be placed. The pusher tube fits into the flange of the stent. Since the stent is 13 cm in this case, a mark "A" will be made on the pusher tube at 12 cm beyond the flange. This will signify the point at the incisors where the distal stent tip first encounters the proximal tumor margin at 25 cm. Mark "B" will be made 10 cm from "A". It will correlate with the distance required to seat the distal flange at 25 cm—the shaft minus the flange is 10 cm (Fig. 4.30).

Just before prosthesis insertion and placement, the 11 mm stabilizing dilator is passed over the guidewire into the mouth and through the tumor into the stomach. The well-lubricated stent and pusher tube are positioned over the stabilizing dilator and advanced through the pharynx. Since this is a relatively large diameter to swallow, there may be some difficulty going though the pharynx and it helps to hyperextend the neck. When mark "A" is at the incisors, the distal stent has reached the proximal margin of the tumor. There may be resistance and

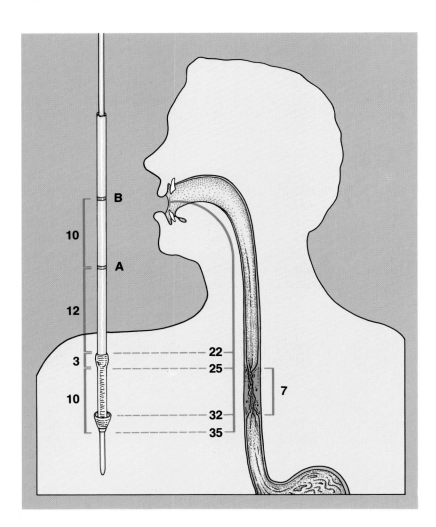

FIGURE 4.30 Pusher tube markings for a 7 cm tumor, the proximal ledge of which is located 25 cm from incisors and the distal ledge at 32 cm. "A" indicates the distance from the distal stent tip to the incisors when the stent is poised at the proximal tumor edge. If the proximal tumor margin is 25 cm from the incisors, as in this example, "A" is 12 cm from the stent flange. "B" denotes the distance from the incisors to the distal stent tip after stent placement. In this case, "B" is 10 cm from "A." The pusher tube is marked by laying it on a flat surface prior to fitting it into the stent flange.

TREATMENT OF ESOPHAGEAL AND OTHER GI CANCERS

firm pressure may be required. Fluoroscopy is useful. A "give" is often appreciated at the time of passage and the pusher tube is advanced until mark "B" is at the incisors. At this point the stent is properly seated (Fig. 4.31). If placement is satisfactory, remove the stabilizing dilator and guidewire.

At this time, the pusher tube is loosened but not withdrawn. It must be pulled back a few cm, so that the suture can be removed. Pull on the ends of each string and remove them one at a time. If removal of the suture causes the stent to move proximally, it can be nudged distally with the pusher tube. A second reason for leaving the pusher tube in place is so that the poststent placement endoscopy can be carried out without having the patient swallow another tube. After the sutures are removed, a small caliber endoscope can be passed inside the pusher tube to confirm proper placement of the stent and to make

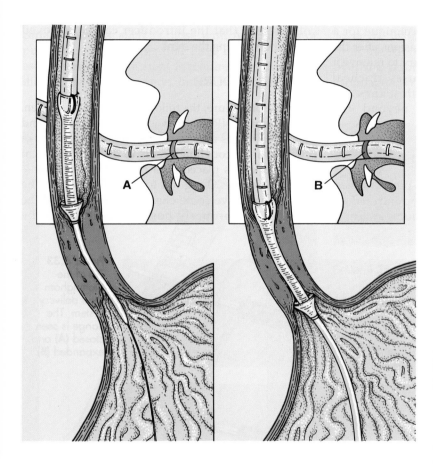

FIGURE 4.31 Pusher tube markings will help assure proper stent placement. Mark "A" will reach the incisors at the point at which distal end of stent reaches the proximal tumor margin. Stent and pusher tube are positioned over outside of stablizing dilator ready for advancement to tumor site. Mark "B" will reach incisors when flange is seated at proximal tumor margin. Pusher tube advances stent into proper placement.

position is correct, the inflating canula is pulled (Fig. 4.37) to inflate the balloon. The combination of air and foam in the balloon sustains enough pressure on the esophageal wall to keep it in place without imparting so much pressure that tissue necrosis will be a problem.

TUMOR AT THE ESOPHAGOGASTRIC JUNCTION

It is easiest to insert stents, and they function best, when the entire shaft lies within the straight segment of the esophagus. Obstructing neoplasms at the esophagogastric (EG) junction may present treatment difficulties whether the intended therapy is a stent or one of the thermal choices. One theoretical concern about violating the EG junction with a prosthesis is that esophageal reflux and possibly aspiration will occur. This concern can usually be addressed by positioning the patient at a 45° angle in bed and by reducing gastric secretion with high doses of an H_2-antagonist or omeprazole. The major practical concern is proper positioning of the stent, so that its tip does not impact against the lesser curve and its position will minimize the likelihood of migration. Ideally, commercially available stents will be made with a bend at the distal margin to deal with these problems. That would also minimize the likelihood of proximal slippage that is likely to occur when a coiled spring is put under tension and has no catch point to

which its distal flange can anchor. Until such a properly molded stent is developed, the best solution is to use a stent 5 to 10 cm longer than that actually required to traverse the tumor. This will usually allows the distal shaft to lie horizontally in the body/antrum of the stomach. In this position, the tip is less likely to be impacted and the tension at the bend point will be reduced.

TUMOR NEAR CRICOPHARYNGEUS

A different problem exists when the tumor is in the cervical esophagus and either invades the upper esophageal sphincter (UES) or requires that the top flange on the stent comes into contact with the UES. There are no easy solutions. First consider whether alternative therapies, such as laser or bipolar coagulation, might be applicable. Also remember that in this area luminal patency cannot be equated with relief of dysphagia, since neuromuscular dysfunction may be associated with the cancer.

If a stent is considered the best option, a few points are worth remembering. Some patients can tolerate a stent placed across the UES without pain, coughing and aspiration, but most cannot. There is no way of predicting which patient will accept it. If a stent is used, choose one with a soft, low profile (flat) upper flange (Fig 4.38). If the tumor itself does not come all the way up to the UES, but the 3 cm upper flange hits

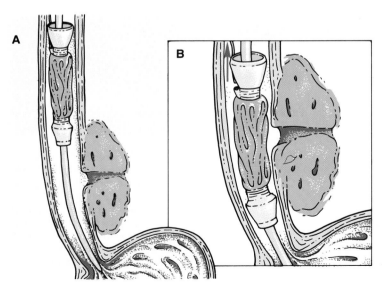
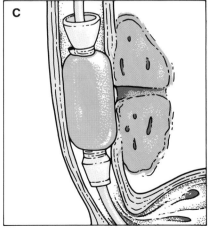

FIGURE 4.37 Stent with cuff deflated is inserted into the esophagus (A). The cannula is pulled when the stent is properly inserted (B). The cuff inflates (C).

it, either use a low profile stent or cut off part of the flange to prevent it from irritating the crico-pharyngeus.

Tumor Overgrowth

On occasion, a stent will function well for weeks or months and then the patient experiences recurrent dysphagia. The problem may be stent obstruction by tumor overgrowth at the proximal or distal end (Fig 4.39). When this occurs, the tumor can usually be debrided by treatment with laser or snare electrocautery.

Although the stents are made of material that is potentially flammable, to date no fires have been reported. A fire would be extremely unlikely, since oxygen concentration is substantially lower than in the situation where endotracheal tubes have ignited when lasers were used to treat pulmonary tumors.

Stent Migration

Migration is the most common difficulty encountered after the stent has been successfully placed (Fig 4.40). Estimates about the incidence vary from 10% to 40%. Most often, the stent migrates proximally.

If the stent is deemed to be the "right stent," it is best to try repositioning it. Replacement is necessary if the chosen stent is:

- Too long; its distal margin is occluded by normal tissue
- Too short; it doesn't fully traverse the tumor.
- Slips because the tension at the esophagogastric junction is too great.

If the stent needs replacement, it can either be removed or pushed into the stomach. A stent that has migrated distally beyond the obstructing neoplasm is

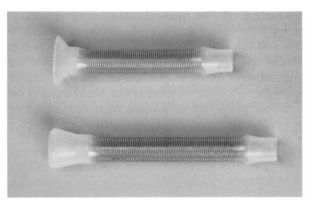

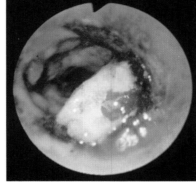

FIGURE 4.39 Endoscopic view shows a tumor obstructing the distal margin of the stent.

FIGURE 4.38 This stent has a low profile, upper flange that is flatter and softer (above) than the upper flange on a standard stent (below).

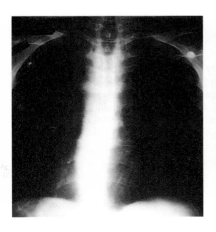
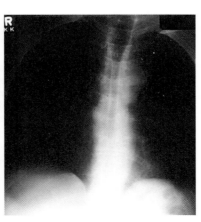

FIGURE 4.40 Radiographs of a patient who experienced stent migration.

functional gastric emptying difficulties and there is often tumor anorexia.

A particularly valuable application of ELT has been for metastatic lesions to the stomach that cause GI bleeding. Whereas ELT has little use for hemorrhages caused by a diffusely friable and hemorrhagic gastric adenocarcinoma or lymphoma, it has proven very beneficial for focal metastasis from breast or renal carcinomas (Fig. 4.42) and malignant melanomas. Laser therapy is more effective than bipolar coagulation or heat probe because it penetrates more deeply. The goal of treatment is to coagulate the feeding tumor vessels and to shrink or obliterate the lesion (Fig. 4.43). Multiple sites may be treated. Lesions less than 5 cm respond best.

One of the most promising conditions for endoscopic therapy is early gastric cancer—either with standard laser therapy or with photodynamic therapy (PDT). As definition of tumor penetration becomes precise and reliable, laser therapy will offer an appealing option to conventional surgery.

COLORECTAL NEOPLASMS

Laser therapy has been used to treat villous adenomas which could not be removed by polypectomy or which recurred after surgery; for residual polyps in the rectal stump after ileorectal anastomoses in patients with familial polyposis, and for obstructing or bleeding tumors in patients who are not operative candidates or who have widespread metastatic disease.

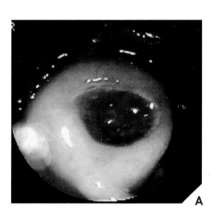 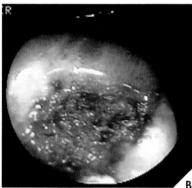

FIGURE 4.42 Renal cell carcinoma metastisizing to the stomach may cause GI bleeding. Endoscopic views before (**A**) and after (**B**) laser therapy.

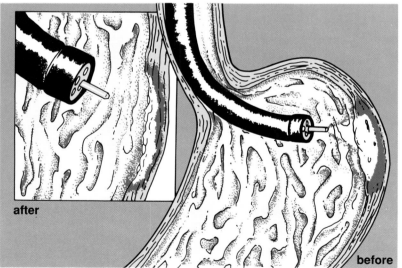

FIGURE 4.43 Endoscopic laser therapy for metastatic lesions have proven to be more successful than bipolar coagulation because it can penetrate deeper.

The treatment of obstructing colorectal tumors is similar to esophageal cancer but a few points are worth stressing. The primary experience is with rectal and low sigmoid tumors. Treatment in other areas is fraught with higher risks and is technically more difficult. If the lumen is almost completely obliterated, dilation with through-endoscope balloon catheters is useful for temporary opening and allows the endoscopist to better assess and treat the luminal pathway (Fig. 4.44). For rectal cancers, it is on occasion easier to use a rigid proctoscope and hand-held laser fiber. If the lesion has advanced to the anal verge, treatment with the Nd:YAG laser is painful and a saddle block may be required. In treating circumferential rectal lesions, one is better off treating only 270° rather than 360° to minimize the risk of rectal stenosis (Fig. 4.45). Patients with rectal tumors are generally more amenable to outpatient treatment than patients with esophageal cancer, who are often more debilitated.

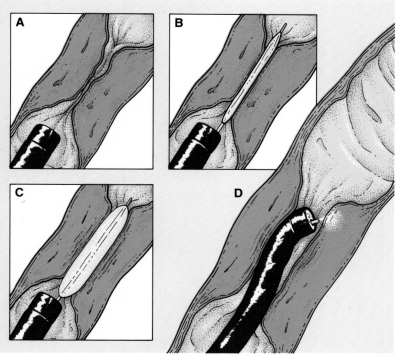

FIGURE **4.44** When the endoscope encounters lumen occluded by tumor in rectosigmoid colon, the endoscope cannot be advanced, and "blind" laser treatment would be risky (**A**). Balloon dilation of obstructed lumen would permit laser therapy. Uninflated balloon exiting from endoscope and passing through narrowed lumen (**B**). Inflated balloon stretching tumor (**C**). Temporary dilation allows endoscope to pass obstructed lumen and map out geography of tumor (**D**). Laser treatment commences at superior margin of tumor.

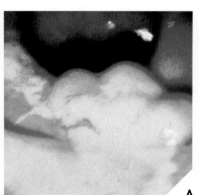
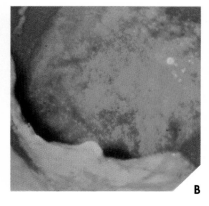

FIGURE **4.45** Nodular, exophytic rectal cancer partially obstructing lumen (**A**). After one session of laser treatment, the lumen is more patent (**B**). (Courtesy of Dr. John Dixon)

REFERENCES

Brunteaud JM, Maunoury V, Cochelard D, et al: Endoscopic laser treatment for rectosigmoid villous adenomas. *Gastroenterology* 1989;97:272.

Earlham R, Cunha-Melo JR: Malignant esophageal stricture: A review of techniques for palliative intubation. *Br J Surg* 1982;69:61.

Fleischer D: Endoscopic laser therapy for esophageal cancer: Present status with emphasis on past and future. *Lasers in Surg Med* 1989;9:6.

Jensen DM, Machicado GM, Randall G, et al: Comparison of low power YAG laser and BICAP tumor probe for palliation of esophageal cancer strictures. *Gastroenterology* 1988;94:1263.

Mellow MH: Endoscopic laser therapy as an alternative to palliative surgery for adenocarcinoma of the rectum—comparison of costs and complications. *Gastrointest Endosc* 1989;35:283.

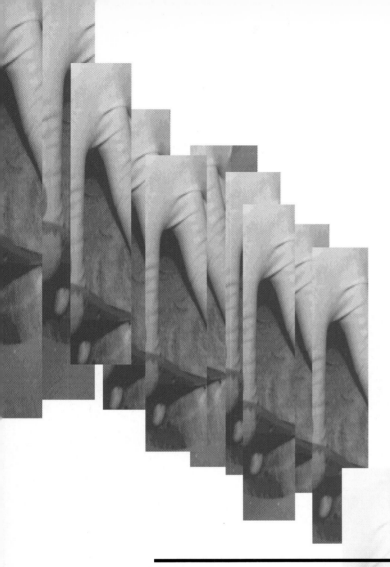

Percutaneous Endoscopic Gastrostomy and Jejunostomy

Jerome D. Waye, MD
Blair S. Lewis, MD

5

Percutaneous Endoscopic Gastrostomy

Introduction

Endoscopically guided percutaneous gastrostomy tube placement was developed in 1980 by Dr. Jeffrey Ponsky. Both techniques and apparatus have evolved rapidly from makeshift collections of urinary and intravenous catheters, to the current choice of three different methods with a variety of commercially available kits.

Technique

The key to percutaneous placement is to have the stomach and the abdominal wall in close apposition without intervening viscera. Therefore, an absolute requirement for percutaneous endoscopic gastrosto-

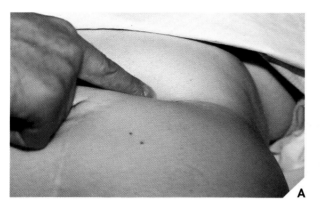

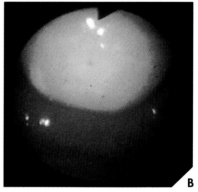

FIGURE 5.1 A finger is placed at the point of maximal transillumination on the abdomen, and pressure is applied (A). The endoscopic image shows a smooth indentation (B).

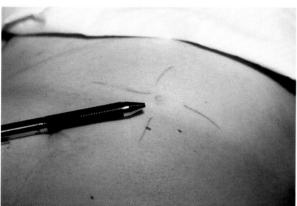

FIGURE 5.2 Skin indentation made with tip of ball-point pen. Ink lines may be removed during skin prep.

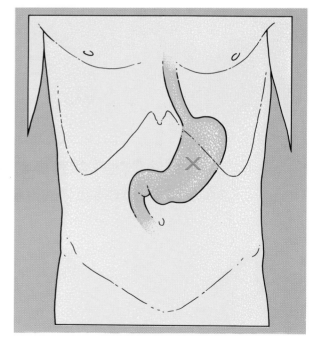

FIGURE 5.3 The point at which the endoscopist notes maximal indentation of the anterior gastric wall is marked to indicate the site for gastrostomy. It may be in the midline and should be more than 2 cm from the lower margin of the left rib cage.

my (PEG) placement is that transillumination through the abdominal wall can be seen with the endoscope in the stomach. Previous concerns that postoperative patients were not candidates for PEG placement, especially following Billroth II resection, have not been borne out.

Antibiotics are usually given prior to the procedure to prevent wound infection. Some authors advocate oral hygiene with an iodinated disinfectant rinse prior to endoscopic passage to decrease the incidence of infection. The procedure is performed with the patient supine. As the risk of aspiration is increased in this position, close attention must be given to the airway.

After standard sedation, a complete EGD is performed. If a PEG is to be placed in a small child or baby, total EGD is not performed as gastric distention with air can lead to diaphragmatic compression causing hypoventilation. Presence of peptic ulcers—gastric or duodenum—during endoscopic examination is not a contraindication to placement of a PEG; however, the puncture site of the PEG should not be through an ulcer bed. A duodenal ulcer with outlet obstruction is a contraindication to PEG.

With the tip in the fundus, the greater and lesser curvatures are identified. The room lights are dimmed to locate the site of transillumination. The new video endoscopes may not provide sufficient light and transillumination may not be possible. However, some endoscopes have a high intensity control that permits light to penetrate the abdominal wall. Exact localiza-

tion of the PEG site is determined by indenting the abdominal wall with the index finger (Fig. 5.1). This maneuver allows the puncture site on the skin to be chosen precisely, since the endoscopist visually verifies the point of maximal indentation. This point is usually found after a few exploratory palpations in the area of transillumination. The chosen site should be on a flat surface of the stomach wall as determined endoscopically. The skin site may be temporarily marked by a firm indentation with the tip of a ball point pen. Simply drawing an "x" or a circle in ink may be insufficient as the skin prep may erase the lines (Fig. 5.2). The endoscopist should maintain eye-contact with the point of maximal indentation since that will be the point through which the stylus will enter the stomach. Some feel that palpation alone without the need for transillumination is sufficient. The ideal site on the abdominal wall is in the left upper quadrant (Fig. 5.3). Within the stomach, a site high in the gastric body is best as this area has no peristaltic contractions. Antral placement can be performed if no other site is found.

PONSKY PERCUTANEOUS ENDOSCOPIC GASTROSTOMY

The skin is prepped and draped (Fig. 5.4). Local injection of lidocaine intracutaneously and subcutaneously at the previously located site anesthestizes the skin and deeper tissues (Fig. 5.5). A 1 cm incision is carried

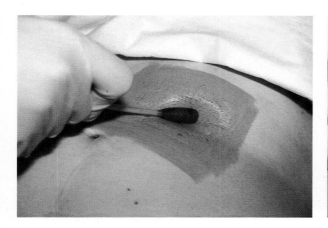

FIGURE 5.4 Typical skin prep over previously identified site.

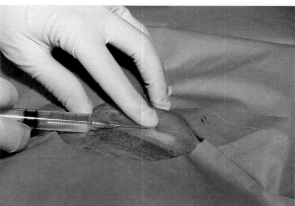

FIGURE 5.5 Injection of local anesthetic agent.

down to the subcutaneous tissues (Fig. 5.6). The risk of bleeding is less from a vertical incision as opposed to a horizontal one. A 1 cm incision aids in avoidance of wound infection by allowing post-procedure drainage of any subcutaneous fluid (Fig. 5.7). The stomach is distended with air. The site is re-identified endoscopically by palpation and an open snare is placed over this point (Fig. 5.8). A sterile long plastic sheathed needle is quickly thust through the incision into the stomach (Fig. 5.9).

In children, the needle is held closer to the tip to avoid inadvertent puncture through the posterior wall with the possibility of aortic laceration. The needle enters the stomach through the open snare loop which is then closed gently (Fig. 5.10). Repositioning the snare may be required to capture the sheathed needle (Fig. 5.11). Entrapment of the needle by the snare secures control and keeps the stomach against the abdominal wall should the patient move or cough.

The needle trocar is removed and a wire loop is advanced through the plastic catheter into the stomach (Fig. 5.12). The snare is opened slightly and lifted off the catheter to encircle the wire loop. The snare is closed completely on the loop (Fig. 5.13). The snare is retracted to the instrument tip and the endoscope is withdrawn pulling the wire loop with it (Fig. 5.14). Once the wire loop exits the mouth, the snare is opened and the wire disengaged. The endoscope is set aside and the snare removed.

Most commerical kits use a knotless technique. The loop on the end of the feeding tube is placed through the wire loop protruding from the mouth—the end of the tube is threaded into the loop on its end. Pulling the tube through its own loop secures the tube to the wire loop protruding from the mouth (Fig. 5.15). One hand is applied firmly on the abdominal wall to prevent excess stretching as the tube traverses the stomach and cutaneous tissues (Fig. 5.16). Pulling the wire

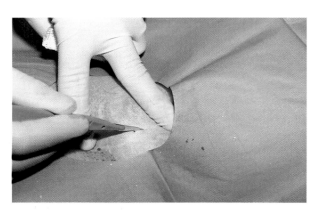

Figure 5.6 A 1 cm vertical incision at the chosen site.

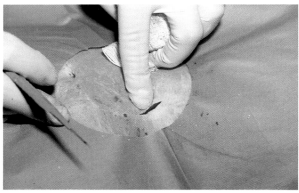

Figure 5.7 Bleeding is less following a vertical incision than one placed horizontally.

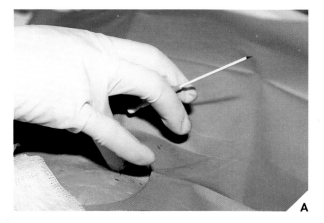

A

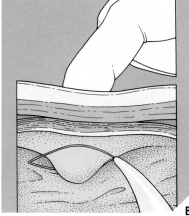

Figure 5.8 To assure proper internal placement of the snare, the abdominal wall site is again palpated with a sterile finger to re-identify the entry site for the sheath and needle.

B

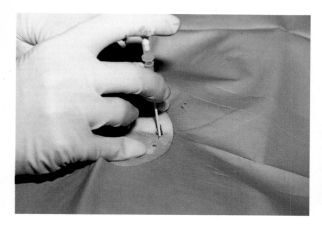
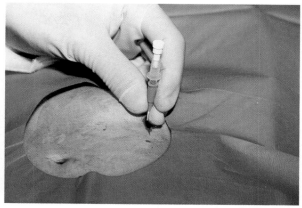

FIGURE 5.9 The sheathed needle is quickly thrust through the incision into the stomach.

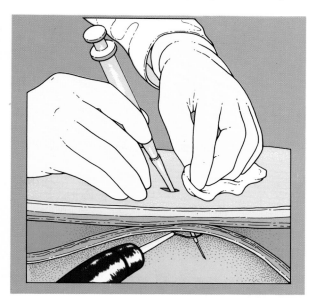

FIGURE 5.10 The sheathed needle enters the stomach through the polypectomy snare which has been carefully positioned under the entry site.

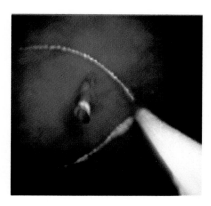

FIGURE 5.11 Endoscopic view of sheathed needle entering the stomach through the snare.

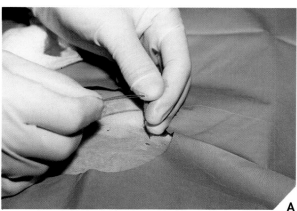

A

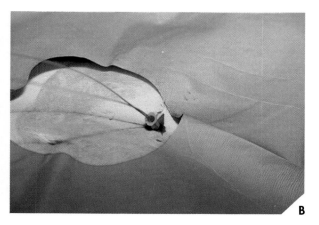

B

FIGURE 5.12 A wire loop is passed through the sheath into the stomach (A). Covering the sheath tip prevents escape of air before the wire loop is inserted (B).

PERCUTANEOUS ENDOSCOPIC GASTROSTOMY AND JEJUNOSTOMY

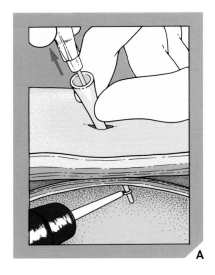

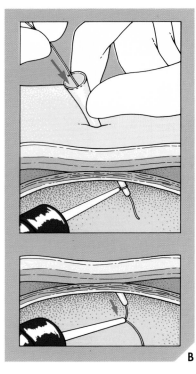

A

B

FIGURE 5.13 The sheath is held in place during needle removal to prevent dislodgment (**A**). The suture is advanced through the sheath directly into the stomach. Simple closure of the snare, after loosening its grip on the sheath, captures the sutures (**B**).

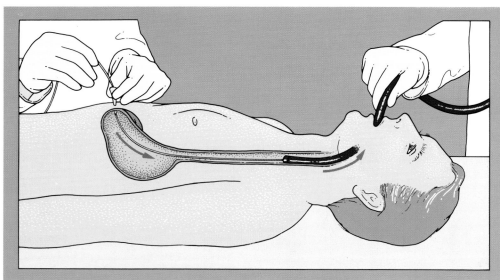

FIGURE 5.14 The endoscope, with the snare and suture retracted into the accessory channel, is withdrawn through the patient's mouth.

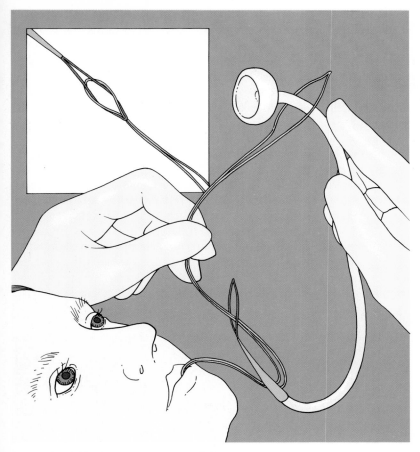

FIGURE 5.15 The knotless technique to attach the feeding tube to the guidewire involves passing the guidewire through the loop at the end of the feeding tube, then placing the bolster of the feeding tube through the guidewire to form a figure "8" knot.

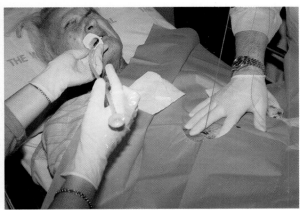

FIGURE 5.16 Firm abdominal pressure is applied as the guidewire is pulled at the skin level, delivering the introducer and feeding tube through the incision.

causes the tube with its built-in dilator to travel down the esophagus into the stomach and out the skin (Fig. 5.17). Although the feeding tube with its tapered end appears to be one piece, the dilator portion is often not firmly attached to the feeding tube. The loop that traverses the dilator, exiting on its tip, is firmly fixed to the long portion of the feeding tube. As the dilating tip may not be tightly affixed to the feeding tube, it should not be pulled upon to assist in passing the apparatus through the abdominal wall, lest the tip disconnect, and leave the blunt end of the feeding tube in the stomach or in the abdominal wall. Pulling the wire alone provides sufficient traction to allow the feeding tube to exit from the skin. When using a commercially made kit with a large intragastric flange, it is necessary to pull enough tube through the skin to prevent airway obstruction. When pulling the dilator section through the skin is difficult, a gentle to-and-fro motion in line with the incision usually delivers the feeding

tube. If the incision is not sufficient to permit egress, it can be enlarged. To prevent lacerating the feeding tube, the scalpel should be held vertically to the skin with the back of the blade touching the feeding tube. A single downward motion of the scalpel into the wound on each side of the feeding tube is usually sufficient to enlarge the incision and allow delivery of the PEG tube.

A second endoscopy is performed to position the internal bolster against the gastric mucosa while an external bolster or cross-bar is slid onto the feeding tube to keep the stomach wall against the parietal peritoneum (Fig. 5.18). Avoidance of excess tension on both the skin and stomach walls is important to avoid pressure necrosis, infection, and tube expulsion. Adequate apposition of the stomach and abdominal walls will be accomplished if the outside bolster is placed 1 to 2 mm from the skin surface while the internal bolster touches the stomach wall (Fig. 5.19).

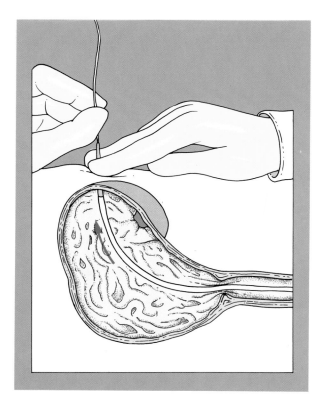

FIGURE 5.17 By pulling the guidewire, the introducer dilates the tract between the gastric and abdominal walls. The introducer is not grasped as it passes through the abdominal wall.

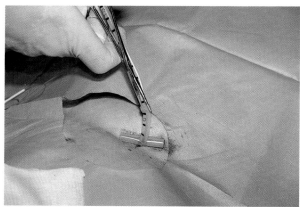

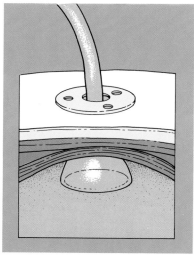

FIGURE 5.18 The external bolster is applied to keep the gastric and abdominal walls in close apposition.

Sacks-Vine Percutaneous Endoscopic Gastrosotomy

The Sacks-Vine technique is presently the most popular gastrostomy. This was the first commercially manufactured gastrostomy kit. The initial advantage of the Sacks-Vine was its greater length, resulting in better "control." The feeding tube could be held at the mouth at the same time as the dilator portion exited the skin. Newer commercially made Ponsky type kits are made of longer feeding tubes that also provide this "control" and the advantage of the Sacks-Vine technique is no longer exclusive. The procedure is essentially the same as the Ponsky technique. Instead of a wire loop passed through the sheath after the puncture, a straight wire is caught by the snare and brought out through the mouth. A stiff long feeding tube with a built-in dilator is then threaded over the guide wire. Holding both ends of the guide wire taut, the tube is then pushed down the esophagus, through the stomach and out through the skin (Fig. 5.20). This technique is called a push PEG, in distinction to the pull PEG of the Ponsky technique.

Russell Percutaneous Endoscopic Gastrostomy

The Russell PEG is a distinct departure from the other two and applies the Seldinger technique to the method. Once the PEG site is chosen and anesthetized, a puncture is made with a long unsheathed needle. A J-tipped guide wire is advanced into the stomach

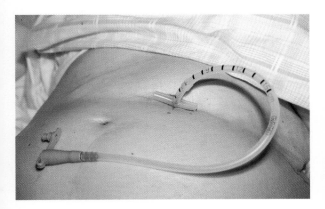

Figure 5.19 No sutures are necessary to maintain the external crossbar in position. The completed PEG may be dressed if desired.

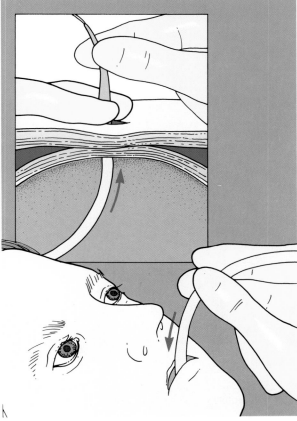

Figure 5.20 In the Sacks-Vine technique, the feeding tube is pushed over a guidewire. It traverses the esophagus and exits through the abdominal wall.

under endoscopic vision (Fig. 5.21). An incision is made alongside the guide wire using a sharp scalpel supplied with the kit. After removal of the guide needle, an introducer with a tight-fitting peel-away sheath is advanced over the wire into the stomach with rapid 180° twisting motions. The introducer is removed and a type of Foley catheter is placed through the sheath into the stomach. After inflation of the balloon, the sheath is peeled away leaving the Foley in place. A disc-shaped cuff is placed around the catheter at skin level to maintain gastric-abdominal wall apposition.

TUBE REMOVAL

Feeding tubes may require replacement. Latex tubes become brittle and cracked and interior bolsters can be eroded by acid. Tubes may become clogged with pills or feeds if not flushed routinely. Some PEGs can be removed percutaneously with gentle traction. While one hand grasps the PEG tube, the other hand maintains pressure on the abdominal wall. The intragastric bumper will compress and be delivered through the skin. Some PEGs with a large intragastric flange cannot be removed percutaneously and must be removed endoscopically. Although PEGs can be

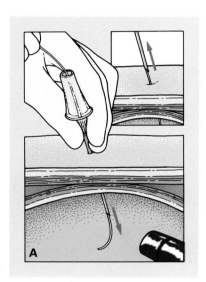

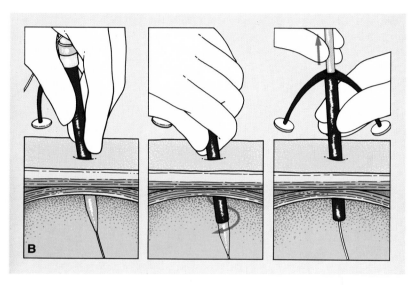

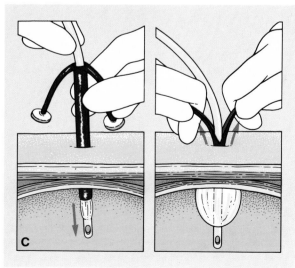

FIGURE 5.21 PEG with a commercial kit. After gastrostomy site is selected, a J-tip guidewire is passed through a needle into the stomach under endoscopic observation. The needle is withdrawn leaving the guidewire in place. A short skin incision is made alongside the guidewire (**A**). A hollow plastic "split sleeve" surrounding a tapered dilator is threaded over the guidewire which is then bent over the top of the entire assembly. Gastric entry is accomplished with a corkscrew twisting motion until the sleeve is seated within the stomach. The introducer and needle are removed (**B**). A feeding catheter is passed through the sleeve. After endoscopic confirmation of its intragastric position, the catheter balloon is inflated. The handles of the split sleeve are pulled apart, peeling it away from the catheter, and leaving the catheter in place for feedings (**C**).

cut at the skin and left to pass naturally, this is not generally accepted because small bowel obstruction and perforation have been reported. To remove a PEG endoscopically, the internal bolster is encircled by an open snare. The external portion of the tube is then advanced into the stomach 5 to 8 cm. The snare is closed on the tubular portion of the PEG. The tube is then cut at the skin level while the intragastric portion is grasped by the snare. The reason for advancing the PEG tube into the stomach and for not grasping the tubing where it joins the bolster is to permit easier removal. The bolster will not be at right angles to the esophagus and will turn and easily traverse the levels of the upper and lower esophageal sphincters (Fig. 5.22). The fibrous tract formed in 2 to 4 weeks between the gastric lumen and the parietal peritoneum closes rapidly and a tube which falls out inadvertently should be replaced rapidly to prevent the need to repeat the entire PEG placement.

CHOICE OF KITS

All of the currently available kits result in a usable percutaneous gastrostomy. The widest selection of tube and bolster sizes are available with the Ponsky type kits. Adult gastrostomy tubes are generally between 20F and 22F in diameter. Pediatric gastrostomy tubes measure 15F to 16F. A 28F gastrostomy tube is available to be used for placement of a large bore jejunostomy tube. Should simultaneous gastric decompression and jejunal feeding be desired, then initial placement with a 28F gastrostomy tube is recommended.

The endoscopist may choose between a percutaneously or endoscopically removable gastrostomy tube. Several manufacturers presently make PEG tubes that are extractable percutaneously. All Russell kits can be removed percutaneously. Percutaneous removal is an advantage for:

• The patient who needs the PEG for short-term nutrition—3 to 6 months.
• An individual in whom a second endoscopy at a later time may prove difficult.

Patients after head and neck surgery are ideal candidates for these kits. The ease of removal makes these tubes poor choices in the uncooperative patient who may pull out the PEG prior to tract formation. Several companies manufacture PEGs that cannot be pulled out accidentally. These tubes are ideal in the elderly or demented patient whose nutritional requirements are deemed to be long-term. In addition to considerations as to the methods of PEG removal, the size and composition of the internal bolster are important. The smaller the internal bolster or the harder the material,

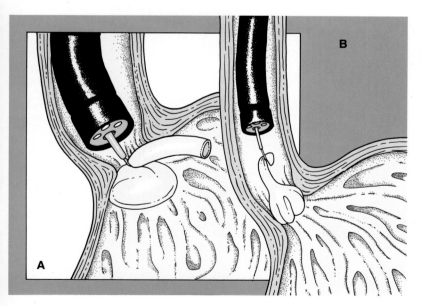

FIGURE 5.22 When removing a PEG endoscopically the tube should be grasped 5 cm to 8 cm from the internal bolster to permit easier removal. Incorrect (A) and correct (B) snare placement are shown.

the greater the risk of gastric pressure necrosis or tube extrusion. The ideal PEG has a nonlatex tube that is long enough to provide control at both ends during insertion with a wide and soft internal bolster. The external bolster should provide easy access for wound cleansing and be relatively flat on the abdominal wall if the patient is to become dressed and is ambulatory.

REPLACEMENT

There are several choices for replacement gastrostomy tubes, none of which require a repeat endoscopy. A standard Foley catheter can be used, but it is long and tube migration may occur since external bolsters are not available. Migration to and blockage of the pylorus or the duodenum may present clinically as gastric out-let obstruction with nausea and vomiting. Short Foley replacement gastrostomy tubes are available with an external bolster preventing migration (Fig. 5.23). The latest option for tube replacement is the so-called "gastrostomy button," offered by several manufacturers (Fig. 5.24). This apparatus has a malecot-type end to hold the tip in the stomach and is available in several lengths to traverse the abdominal wall (Fig. 5.25). The feeding port is covered with a screw or a snap top. The buttons barely protrude above skin level, and are equipped with a flap valve to prevent reflux. They are ideal for a fully functioning patient who does not want tubing protruding under clothing. The original PEG can be removed in 4 to 6 weeks after insertion and the button may be inserted at that time.

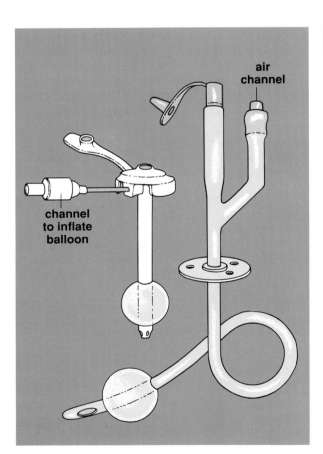

FIGURE 5.23 Foley replacement tubes are shorter then urinary catheters to avoid distal migration and resultant obstruction of the pylorus or duodenum.

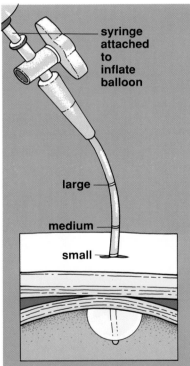

FIGURE 5.24. Low profile devices come in several lengths. The tract should be measured prior to selecting the appropriate replacement tube. A thin Foley is advanced through the tract and its balloon inflated. The tube is then withdrawn to seat the balloon on the internal gastric wall. Markings on the thin Foley are then used to measure the tract length.

Percutaneous Endoscopic Jejunostomy

Intrajejunal tube feeding can be accomplished by positioning a catheter in the small bowel through a PEG. Gastric decompression and simultaneous jejunal feeding is also possible using different sized PEG and PEJ tubing (Fig. 5.26). Several commercially available kits are available. Generally all manufacturers sell PEJ tubes that can fit through their gastrostomy tubes. It is not necessary to use matching kits for this insertion as 8F to 12F jejunostomy tubes can fit through 20F diameter PEG tubes.

Technique

In general, a long weighted tube is passed through a PEG and endoscopically positioned in the small bowel. Initially a wide caliber PEG is placed and secured as usual. The PEG tube is cut 8 cm to 10 cm from the skin and a jejunostomy tube (J-tube)

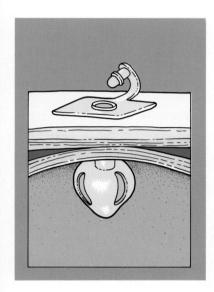

Figure 5.25 Many low profile replacement devices use deformable internal malecot-type ends to hold the tube in place.

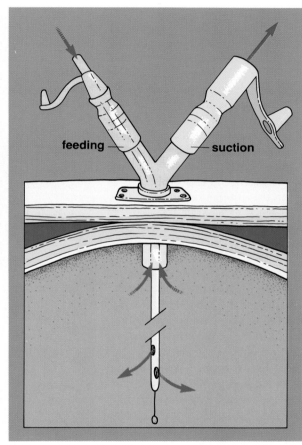

feeding — suction

Figure 5.26 Concomitant jejunal feedings and gastric decompression may be accomplished by passing a jejunal tube thinner than the gastrostomy tube through the latter. Gastric secretions may then exit through the gastrostomy tube while jejunal feedings are performed.

advanced into the stomach through the gastrostomy tube (Fig. 5.27). The endoscope is used to position the J-tube in the small bowel (Fig. 5.28). Most jejunostomy tubes have weighted tips and stiffening stylets to counteract the tendancy of the jejunal tube to be pulled back from its desired location as the endoscope is withdrawn. The PEG tube must be clamped after it is cut to prevent gastric deflation. The tube is unclamped as the J-tube is advanced until it protrudes through the PEG orifice internally. The PEG tubing with the indwelling J-tube is then reclamped to allow insufflation.

All J-tubes have a suture at the end to facilitate placement. The suture on the tip of the PEJ is grasped close to the feeding tube by a biopsy forceps without a central spike. Entrapment of the suture onto the center spike may interfere with its subsequent release. The forceps and suture are withdrawn to the endoscope tip before advancing the scope into the jejunum. Because there is no visibility without distention the PEG must be repeatedly unclamped as the J-tube is advanced then reclamped to facilitate inflation. Gentle traction must be applied to the PEG tube as it protrudes from the skin whenever the endoscope and J-tube are advanced into the duodenum since friction between the two tubes tends to separate the stomach from the abdominal wall. A gastric leak or large amount of pneumoperitoneum can ensue if traction is not applied to the PEG tube.

Deep placement beyond the ligament of Treitz is necessary. Since a gastroscope does not provide sufficient length for J-tube placement, a pediatric colonoscope is usually employed to allow intubation beyond the ligament of Treitz. The J-tube must be kept straight from its entrance site at the PEG to its tip within the small bowel. Excess J-tube looping within the stomach will invariably lead to failure as the tube falls back upon endoscope withdrawal. The loop may be removed by pulling the J-tube out of the PEG while the closed forceps holds the suture on the end of the tube. Once within the jejunum, the biopsy forceps is pushed forward and opened releasing the J-tube. The J-tube and its stylet are held firmly as the endoscope is removed by freeing the controls and rapidly withdrawing. Most of the small bowel feeding tubes have weighted tips and holes spaced along several inches

proximal to the weighted area. If the tip only reaches the second or third portion of the duodenum, the last feeding hole will still be within the stomach and intragastric feeding will be delivered. Once the J-tube is sited, the amount of tension at the PEG site must be reassessed since leaving the same amount of tension as applied during the PEG placement can lead to pressure necrosis and extrusion. All patients should have an x-ray following PEG placement to assure that kinking and malposition have not occurred.

CHOICE OF PERCUTANEOUS ENDOSCOPIC JEJUNOSTOMY TUBES

A variety of jejunostomy tube sizes are commercially available. Smaller PEJ tubes—between 8F to 10F—tend to clog easily and can kink. Larger bore jejunostomy tubes are generally recommended. Twelve French tubes tend to remain straight and patent longer than the thinner tubes. If gastric decompression is desired,

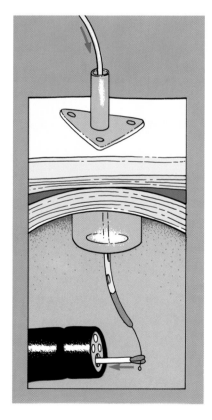

FIGURE 5.27 An orally passed endoscope grasps the jejunostomy tube with attached suture as it is advanced through the gastrostomy tube.

placement of a large bore jejunostomy tube through a 20F or 22F PEG will not work. A 28F large bore PEG tube will be required to allow simultaneous gastric decompression and jejunal feeding. This combination of drainage and feeding occurs in patients with known high gastric residuals either due to functional abnormalities of gastric motility or to partially obstructing tumors. Simultaneous gastric decompression may lower the risk of aspiration in patients receiving PEJ feedings.

FOLLOW-UP

Initially, a dressing may be applied over the gastrostomy site but is not necessary. Daily cleansing with peroxide can lower the incidence of wound infection. Sutures are not used to maintain the position of most external bolsters. By the second day the external bolster should be loosened somewhat to lower the risk of pressure necrosis and extrusion of the intragastric component. A space of 1 to 2 mm between the abdominal wall and the external crossbar will prevent pressure necrosis.

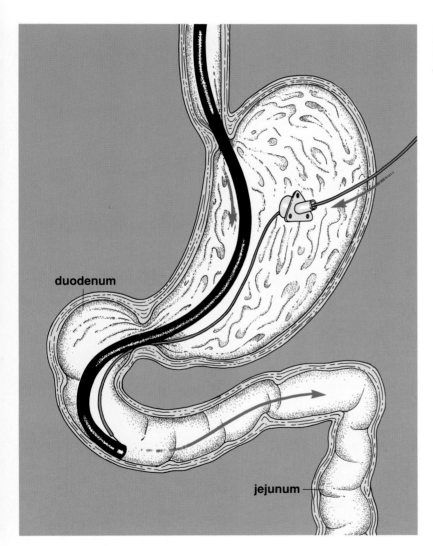

FIGURE 5.28 The endoscope holding the jejunostomy tube is advanced into the jejunum. An x-ray should be obtained prior to starting feedings.

duodenum

jejunum

Enteral Feedings

Depending on the prior condition of the patient, tube feedings may be started immediately or after a period of 24 hrs (Fig. 5.29). Most patients being considered for the placement of a gastrostomy have been fed via nasogastric tubes prior to PEG. For these patients, feedings should be given in the usual amount 24 hrs after the gastrostomy tube has been placed.

In patients who have not received nasogastric nutrition supplements prior to PEG, the rapid introduction of tube feeding may cause diarrhea. Present recommendations are to instill full strength feedings at a slow rate and increase this rate over several days. Full strength iso-osmotic feedings are begun by a slow drip pump technique at a rate of 25 mL/hr increasing to 50 mL/hr the following day. The infusion rate is slowly increased by 25 mL/hr to obtain full nutritional support. It is then possible to progress from a pump delivery system to bolus feeds using gravity bags.

Some blenderized foods may be given through the gastrostomy, but must be liquid in consistency. Clogging of the tube can be prevented with proper care after each feeding. Warm tap water, 50 cc, should be rinsed through the tube via a syringe or gravity bag. Tablets or capsules should be dissolved prior to their instillation if possible but crushing is adequate in most circumstances. All medications must be flushed through the tube after each dose.

Complications

The overall morbidity for PEG is less than 10%. There is a 3% incidence of major complications such as sepsis, inadvertent puncture of another viscus, or laparotomy. Minor complications occur in about 7% of PEG patients. The most frequent minor complication is wound infection which may respond to local treatment, such as peroxide cleansing 3 times daily, antibiotics, or circumstomal drainage. Other complications include leak into the peritoneal cavity because of tube dislodgment, inadvertent removal of the tube and transient fever.

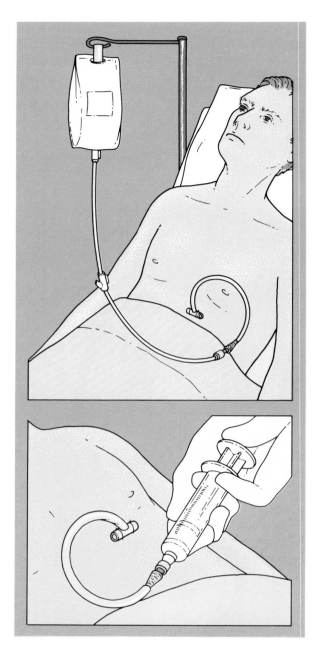

FIGURE 5.29 Percutaneous endoscopic gastrostomy feeding may be given by slow drip method or by bolus via a large syringe.

REFERENCES

Mamel JJ: Percutaneous endoscopic gastrostomy. *Am J Gastroenterol* 1989;84:703.

Miller RE, Winkler WP, Kotler DP: The Russell percutaneous endoscopic gastrostomy: Key technical steps. *Gastrointest Endosc* 1988;34:339.

Ponsky JL, Gauderer MWL: Percutaneous endoscopic gastrostomy: Indications, limitations, techniques, and results. *World J Surg* 1989;13:165.

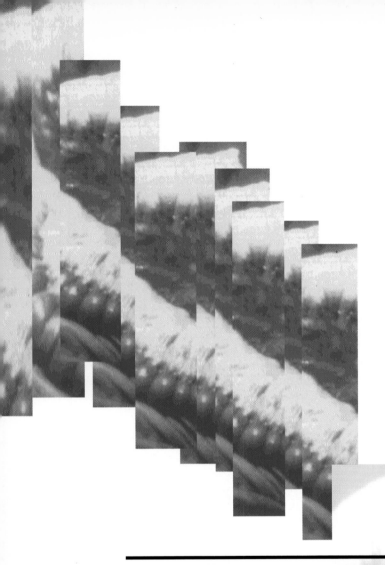

Techniques of Enteroscopy

6

Blair S. Lewis, MD
Jerome D. Waye, MD

INTRODUCTION

Endoscopy of the small bowel is especially useful in the evaluation and treatment of patients with obscure GI bleeding. There are three accepted methods available to endoscopically evaluate the small intestine: push enteroscopy, sonde enteroscopy, and intraoperative enteroscopy. Each has its own advantages and disadvantages. Of the three, the easiest and most rapid is push enteroscopy, which can be performed by anyone trained in upper GI endoscopy.

Sonde and intraoperative enteroscopy are tedious and usually reserved for investigation of patients with melena or positive fecal occult blood testing and iron deficiency anemia. These patients often require multiple blood transfusions. In this group of patients previous evaluations with EGD, colonoscopy, and small bowel x-ray series have failed to determine the site of blood loss.

Although the majority of enteroscopies are performed for obscure bleeding, other indications include evaluation of an x-ray abnormality of the small intestine and the evaluation of Crohn's disease. The yield for finding pathology is low when the procedure is performed for nonbleeding indications such as chronic abdominal pain or weight loss.

PUSH ENTEROSCOPY

Push enteroscopy, advancing a long endoscope into the small intestine during upper intestinal endoscopy, is also termed deep upper endoscopy, extended esophagogastroduodenoscopy, or enteroscopy. Although a pediatric colonoscope is usually used, a standard colonoscope is acceptable. Sterilization is not necessary and a thoroughly clean, disinfected instrument may be used safely.

TECHNIQUE

A standard-size colonoscope, because of its wide diameter, may be difficult to pass through the cricopharynx, but intubation of the pylorus is easily accomplished. Long and relatively narrow scopes utilizing a designated overtube are available for push enteroscopy but are not popular at the present time.

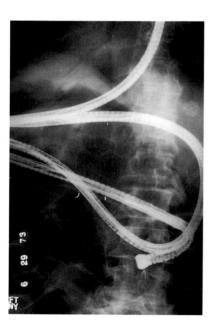

FIGURE 6.1
An orally passed pediatric colonoscope with its tip 60 cm beyond the ligament of Treitz.

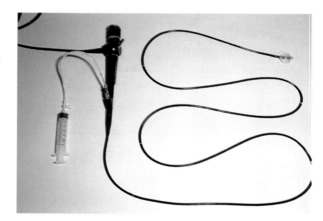

FIGURE 6.2 The small bowel enteroscope with its balloon inflated.

The tip of any long instrument can often be passed to a depth 60 cm beyond the ligament of Treitz (Fig. 6.1). Gentle pressure permits scope advance although a loop invariably forms in the stomach. Because of discomfort as the loop in the stomach distends the greater curvature, an increased amount of sedation may be necessary for the performance of push enteroscopy. The multiple angulations of the small bowel cause difficulty in locating and examining the lumen. A combination of extreme tip deflections and pulling the instrument back will permit identification of the lumen. If deep intubation cannot be achieved, external splinting can be useful: This refers to the technique of deep palpatory pressure on the abdomen to reduce the size of loop formation. The technique is to apply abdominal pressure over the greater curvature of the stomach after reducing the intragastric loop. Upon withdrawal of the endoscope, intravenous glucagon can help to evaluate the small intestine by reducing its motility.

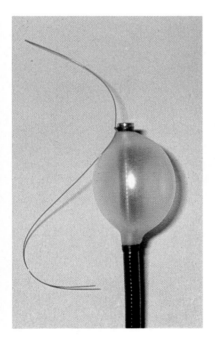

FIGURE 6.3 The balloon at the end of the enteroscope aids in initial placement and eventual passage. A suture is affixed to the tip, used in its placement within the jejunum.

Push enteroscopy is useful to evaluate patients who have obscure gastrointestinal bleeding with yields from 13% to 46% in several series. Fulguration of bleeding sites and polypectomy can be accomplished during the examination. BICAP, heater probe, or hot biopsy forceps can be used safely within the small intestine. During cauterization of vascular ectasias, glucagon should not be used initially because cessation of peristalsis causes pooling of blood and wash effluent that will interfere with visualization. Glucagon may be given after the bleeding site is identified. Active bleeding may be stopped with a submucosal injection using a standard sclerotherapy needle and 1 cc to 5 cc of 1-10,000 epinephrine solution. The volume of injected fluid in interstitial tissue increases the distance between the mucosa and serosa, allowing safe cautery with any thermal device.

SONDE ENTEROSCOPY

Sonde enteroscopy, also termed small bowel enteroscopy, is a nonsurgical method for endoscopy of the small bowel.

TECHNIQUE

The instrument, the SIF-SW, is 9 feet long, has a diameter of 5 mm and a forward 120° angle of view (Fig. 6.2). The small scope allows transnasal passage and the flexibility enables it to transverse the multiple bends and loops of the small bowel. Peristalsis propels the instrument through the intestine and examination is performed during withdrawal. There are two 1 mm internal channels. One is to insufflate a balloon at the instrument tip that acts as a bolus for peristaltic action and also serves to anchor the enteroscope within the small bowel during the initial placement (Fig. 6.3). During endoscope withdrawal, the inflated balloon creates resistance that prevents its excessively rapid removal. The other channel permits insufflation of air to distend the small bowel lumen. The channels are too small to permit passage of any therapeutic instrument or allow suction of luminal contents.

The latex cylinder balloon can be used for an average of 10 examinations. To ensure that the latex cylinder does not lose air it must be meticulously hand-tied onto the instrument. A 3-O silk tie is snugly wrapped for 6 non-overlapping revolutions on the proximal end approximately 3.0 cm from the metal tip. It may be placed in the shallow impression created by the previous suture. The shape of the inflated balloon will be a symmetrical sphere only when the cylinder has been attached with a small amount of linear tension. To achieve this, the free end of the balloon is gently pulled 1 cm to 2 cm beyond the tip of the enteroscope and held in that position by a clamp. Another 3-O silk is tied in the machined metal groove at the endoscope tip and the excess balloon trimmed away. A prolene 2-O suture is threaded through the horizontal hole in the enteroscope's tip and held in place by a knot. This blue suture is used as a handle to pull the small bowel enteroscope through the pylorus by the push enteroscope. Integrity of the balloon should be tested by water immersion after filling with 20 cc air.

Passage of the small bowel enteroscope through the nose is similar to the technique of nasogastric tube placement. Placing the enteroscope through the cricopharynx is facilitated by active swallowing by the unsedated patient.

The blunt-tipped 15F enteroscope will be painful as it traverses the sensitive intranasal mucosa and local anesthesia is required. With the patient supine, the nostrils are anesthetized with cotton tipped wooden applicator sticks soaked in 2% tetracaine (Figs. 6.4, 6.5). The 15 cm stick is advanced until it touches the posterior nasopharynx—usually at a distance of 10 cm from the nares—after which 1 cc of tetracaine is dripped down the applicator stick. The bitter-tasting liquid is swallowed to anesthetize the nasopharynx and the posterior oropharynx. Adequate anesthesia is provided in about 5 min. After removing the applicator stick, the small bowel enteroscope is advanced transnasally into the stomach. To assist in localization, the enteroscope is marked with a white bar every 50 cm. The enteroscope is advanced to the first white mark on the shaft so its tip is in the fundus.

Passive passage of the small bowel enteroscope through the pylorus may be a major rate-limiting factor in enteroscopy. This is circumvented by actively placing the tip of the enteroscope beyond the ligament of Treitz. Since the small-diameter instrument is too flexible to be pushed through the pylorus, the placement is facilitated by using a carrier instrument with tip deflection capability.

Once the enteroscope tip is in the stomach, standard sedation for upper intestinal endoscopy is admin-

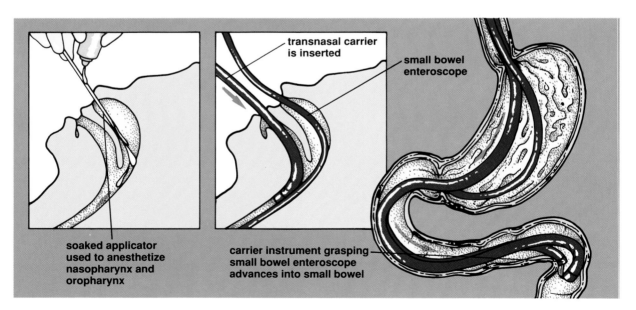

transnasal carrier is inserted

small bowel enteroscope

soaked applicator used to anesthetize nasopharynx and oropharynx

carrier instrument grasping small bowel enteroscope advances into small bowel

Figure 6.4 Technique for placement of small bowel enteroscope.

TECHNIQUES OF ENTEROSCOPY

istered intravenously and the patient is turned to the left lateral decubitis position. A long endoscope used for push enteroscopy is passed orally alongside the small bowel enteroscope (Fig. 6.6). The opportunity should be taken to perform a complete EGD with the push enteroscope, as well as a full push enteroscopy, prior to placing the SIF-SW within the small bowel. The use of the push enteroscope allows greater visibility than is possible with the sonde enteroscope. If definitive pathology such as a small bowel tumor is found, small bowel enteroscopy can be deferred.

After completion of push enteroscopy, the instrument is withdrawn to the gastric fundus. The SIF-SW is seen, and under direct vision through the push enteroscope the sonde scope is advanced until its tip rests in the antrum. A biopsy forceps, with the center spike removed to avoid lacerating the balloon, is advanced through the push enteroscope to grasp the prolene suture as close as possible to the SIF-SW tip (Fig. 6.7). Grasping the suture near the instrument head provides greater ability to advance the SIF-SW tip in front of the push enteroscope while within the small intestine.

In the presence of a large hiatal hernia, the SIF-SW tip may curl within the hiatal sac. The suture can be grasped within the sac to carry the SIF-SW through the diaphragmatic hiatus under direct vision.

With the forceps of the long endoscope holding the SIF-SW suture, the pylorus is approached by usual endoscopic techniques while advancing the shaft of the sonde enteroscope through the nose. The forceps holding the suture is advanced through the pylorus carrying the enteroscope tip with it. An attempt to pull the SIF-SW through the pylous behind the long endoscope may be thwarted because the enteroscope tip tends to catch on the pyloric lip.

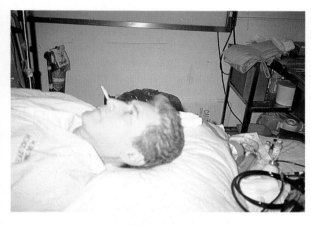

FIGURE 6.5 Tetracaine soaked pledgets are placed in the nostrils to provide topical anesthesia prior to enteroscope passage.

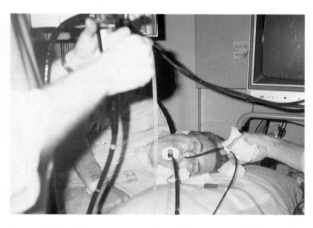

FIGURE 6.6 Both enteroscopes have been passed. The push enteroscope is placed orally while the sonde instrument is transnasal.

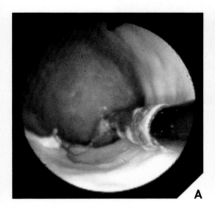

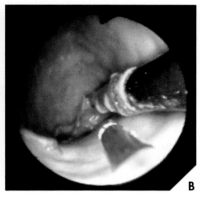

A

B

FIGURE 6.7 The sonde enteroscope lying within the antrum (A). The proline suture is grasped by a biopsy forceps extended from the push enteroscope (B).

Once the forceps and the SIF-SW tip are in the duodenal bulb, the push enteroscope is advanced through the pylorus. As the long scope is advanced, the biopsy forceps with the suture is retracted to avoid trauma to the duodenal bulb. The long endoscope, carrying the small bowel enteroscope, is then advanced to the descending duodenum. When a luminal view is obtained as the push enteroscope enters the descending duodenum, the forceps are again advanced to place the SIF-SW tip in view. The SIF-SW must also be advanced at the nostril to provide slack within the stomach. Without this slack, the SIF-SW will spring backwards into the stomach once the suture is released. Repetition of this series of movements—advance the push enteroscope, advance the forceps and the SIF-SW, advance the SIF-SW at the nostril—continues until the push enteroscope is inserted as deeply as possible. When pulling back on the push enteroscope to find lumen, the SIF-SW is held at the nostril to keep the intragastric portion of the SIF-SW in position.

Upon deep insertion of both scopes into the small bowel, the forceps is extended to visualize the SIF-SW tip. The forceps is opened, releasing the SIF-SW, and withdrawn. The balloon at the SIF-SW tip is inflated. The normal volume of air instilled is 17 to 20 cc (Fig. 6.8). When withdrawing the long endoscope, it is always necessary for the endoscopic assistant to hold the SIF-SW at the nostril to avoid simultaneous withdrawal of the enteroscope from the force of friction. The long endoscope is withdrawn into the stomach using short, jerking motions after loosening the control locks. A full luminal view is not attempted during this phase, as it is important to avoid dislodging the SIF-SW.

With the long endoscope in the stomach, an assessment must be made of the intragastric portion of the small bowel enteroscope shaft. If the SIF-SW is taut along the lesser curvature, the SIF-SW must be advanced through the nostril until there is slack across the greater curvature of the stomach. Loops, if present, should be removed by withdrawing the small bowel enteroscope. Loops that form within the posterior pharynx must also be removed.

The integrity of the balloon is checked by removing a small amount of air and then replacing it. The pressure within the balloon can be readily perceived during this maneuver. The patient assumes a supine position and may be sent to the endoscopy recovery room.

The enteroscope must be periodically advanced into the stomach during its passage through the small bowel (Fig. 6.9). The length of the enteroscope, its flexibility, the limited strength of peristalsis, and friction in the nasopharynx and esophagus, all require that an excess of the enteroscope be present within the stomach. Peristalsis, pulling on the inflated balloon, can draw the slack small bowel enteroscope shaft from the stomach into the small bowel, but it is not sufficient to pull any length of scope from outside the nose. On the other hand, excessive looping within the stomach will halt forward progress. There is a technique for physicians, gastrointestinal nurses, or assistants to gauge the proper length of shaft to be placed in the stomach. This method requires that the enteroscope be withdrawn from the nose until slight tension is felt as the enteroscope becomes taut along the lesser curvature. After applying lubrication, the enteroscope is then advanced until resistance is again felt. This represents the shaft bowing along the greater curvature of the stomach. This maneuver is repeated every 30 to 45 min. Excess stomach coiling may result if an assistant merely advances a predetermined length of scope into the nose at fixed time intervals.

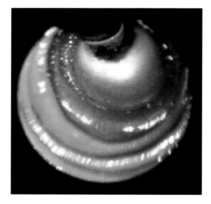

FIGURE 6.8
The sonde enteroscope within the jejunum with its balloon inflated.

Once the entire endoscope is in the patient, or advancement ceases for two successive hours, an x-ray is taken or the patient is fluoroscoped (Fig. 6.10). An arbitrary time limit of 8 hours may be employed as this generally coincides with the working day of the endoscopy unit. Reasons for non-passage include obstructive lesions, small bowel adhesions, and poor peristalsis. Adjusting the balloon size either smaller or larger by 3 cc to 5 cc may aid in passage. When passage is impeded, water-soluble contrast media can be injected through the endoscope's air channel to obtain a limited contrast study of the bowel (enteroclysis) just distal to the arrested tip.

Instrument withdrawal does not require fluo-

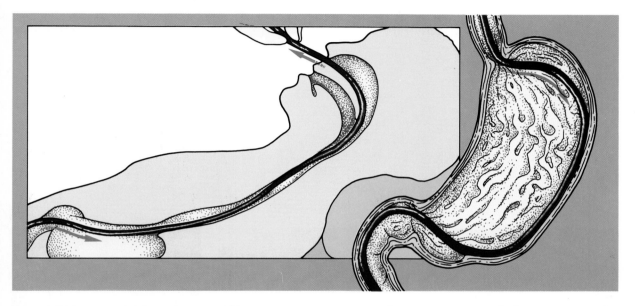

FIGURE 6.9 Maneuvers by the assistant to aid in enteroscope advance at intervals. The shaft is pulled backwards to remove any excess gastric loop. Gentle resistance indicates it is resting on the lesser curvature of the stomach. The instrument is then advanced.

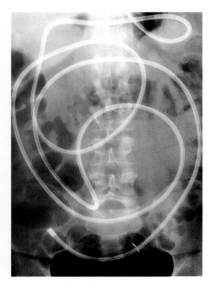

FIGURE 6.10 An x-ray showing complete intubation of the enteroscope to the ileocecal valve.

roscopy or sedation. The SIF-SW is attached to a light source for the first time in the procedure. Air is insufflated using either a hand pump from a rigid sigmoidoscope set or a dedicated air pump. The lumen may not be readily visualized, even though distended with air, and palpation is used to push the bowel into position. There is no tip deflection capability with a small bowel enteroscope and abdominal palpation increases the view by pushing the small bowel into the path of the enteroscope or vice versa. Air insufflation is kept to a minimum, since over-distention can limit abdominal palpation and result in patient discomfort. Once an area has been examined, the balloon is deflated and abdominal pressure is applied to slide the scope cephalad. When pressure fails to be useful, tension is applied at the nostril. The balloon is always deflated during shaft withdrawal to limit pleating of the bowel on the enteroscope. Pleating may lead to rapid unraveling of the bowel off the endoscope tip, leaving a portion of the lumen uninspected. Because of bowel angulation,

lack of tip deflection and the tendency for the scope to spring back rapidly, at best, about 75% of the bowel length traversed is seen during small bowel enteroscopy.

Traction at the nose is applied only until a small amount of retrograde motion at the tip is observed. Abdominal pressure is then applied to increase luminal view and move the enteroscope tip. Balloon inflation can be performed rapidly with air to hold the enteroscope tip in place and to increase the luminal view by bringing the tip away from the wall. Inflation may also be helpful to carry the endoscope forward several inches for reinspection of an area. The process of palpation, balloon deflation, nasal traction, and palpation (with or without balloon inflation), is repeated over and over again. When the tip has been withdrawn to within 100 cm of the nostril, torque applied to the shaft can increase the luminal view. Transmission of torque to the tip is not possible when loops are present in the stomach or small bowel. The scope is delivered through the nostril at the end of the

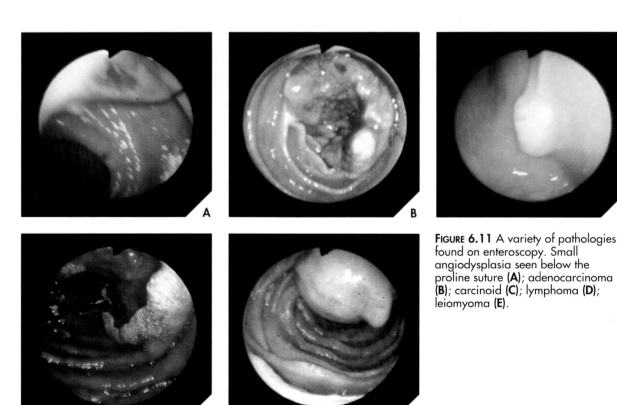

FIGURE 6.11 A variety of pathologies found on enteroscopy. Small angiodysplasia seen below the proline suture (A); adenocarcinoma (B); carcinoid (C); lymphoma (D); leiomyoma (E).

TECHNIQUES OF ENTEROSCOPY

examination, being careful that the balloon is completely deflated as it passes through the pylorus, esophagus, pharynx, and nose. The withdrawal phase lasts approximately 30 to 45 min (Fig. 6.11).

If pathology is found during withdrawal, its general vicinity can be estimated. The instrument is marked every 50 cm for a total of five marks. During withdrawal the first mark places the tip just beyond the pylorus. The second mark indicates the tip is within the proximal jejunum. The third mark generally indicates the distal jejunum, the fourth proximal ileum, and the fifth distal ileum. Even with x-ray control, the localization during withdrawal is approximate and the marks provide only a general guide to tip location. Mucosal landmarks may also be used for localization. The ileal surface is flat with few, short folds (valvulae conniventes) and a vascular pattern is often visible. As the instrument moves cephalad, the folds increase in number and height. In the upper small bowel, where folds become more numerous and more prominent, the mucosal surface in the valleys between the folds is seen less well and the vascular pattern is less apparent.

INTRAOPERATIVE ENDOSCOPY

Intraoperative enteroscopy can provide almost complete visualization of the intestine. With the patient anesthetized, a clean colonoscope is passed orally into the stomach (Fig. 6.12). A standard colonoscope may be difficult to negotiate through the cricopharynx, but the increased length will be necessary for complete examination of the small intestine. The anesthesiologist may be required to deflate the endotracheal tube to allow the scope to advance beyond the cricopharynx. If possible, the tip of the instrument should be at the proximal jejunum prior to opening the abdomen. The intact abdominal wall confines the size of the intragastric loop allowing the instrument to be more easily advanced around the ligament of Treitz. Should intubation be started after the abdomen is open, it may be necessary for the surgeon to cup the duodenal bulb with the left hand and the greater curvature of the stomach with the right hand to confine the loop in the instrument.

An enterotomy to place the endoscope directly into the bowel, without or without a sleeve, is not routine practice due to the possibility of postoperative abdominal infection.

Upon opening the abdomen, a noncrushing clamp is placed over the distal ileum to prevent undesirable distention of the large bowel with air, a nuisance when attempting to close the abdominal incision. Once beyond the ligament of Treitz, the surgeon can grasp the instrument and advance it through the small bowel, holding a 5 cm to 10 cm segment of small bowel in front of the instrument for the endoscopist to evaluate. After affirmation of normalcy, that segment is pleated onto the colonoscope. Concomitant passage of a nasogastric tube is recommended since overinflation of the stomach with air can lead to multiple mucosal lacerations.

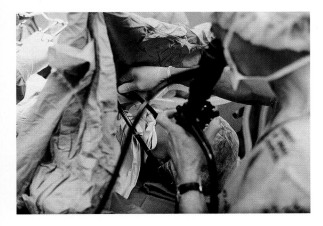

FIGURE 6.12 Intraoperative enteroscopy is performed with oral passage of a colonoscope.

The major indication for this procedure is identification and resection of bleeding sites in patients with obscure GI bleeding. Intraoperative endoscopic fulguration or polypectomy of detected lesions can limit the amount of bowel removed; however, surgical resection of a segment containing an arteriovenous malformation (AVM) is more definitive. It may be useful for finding and removing small bowel polyps or to guide a surgeon through dense adhesions. Visualization within the small bowel is limited if the patient has recently bled or is actively bleeding at the time of endoscopy. Prolonged postoperative ileus has been described in some patients secondary to the small bowel trauma.

Intraoperative enteroscopy is not an easy examination and requires a great deal of patience. Examination of the bowel should be carried out during intubation, as excessive trauma to the bowel from pleating will cause multiple crush artifacts rendering interpretation difficult upon endoscope withdrawal. With this method it may occasionally not be possible to reach the terminal ileum using 165 cm instruments. Enterotomy can be considered at these times. When a lesion is found at intraoperative endoscopy, the surgeon marks the area by placing a suture through the serosa (Figs. 6.13, 6.14). The endoscope is then advanced until the entire intestine is examined (Fig. 6.15). After the endoscope has been withdrawn, and all the excess gas removed, the surgeon can determine the location and extent of resection based on groupings of the serosal ligatures.

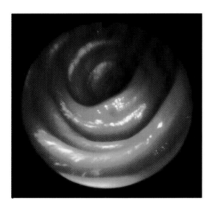

FIGURE 6.13 An angiodysplasia found at intraoperative enteroscopy. Note the room lights shining through the bowel wall.

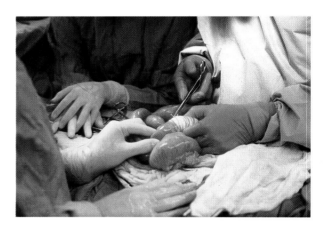

FIGURE 6.14 Upon finding a lesion endoscopically, a suture marks the site on the serosa.

FIGURE 6.15 The entire small bowel has been pleated on a colonoscope passed orally.

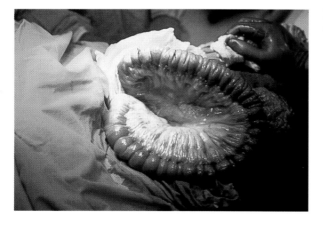

REFERENCES

Bowden T, Hooks V, Mansberger A: Intraoperative gastrointestinal endoscopy. *Ann Surg* 1980;191:680.

Lewis BS, Waye JD: Small bowel enteroscopy in 1988: Pros and cons. *Am J Gastroenterol* 1988;83:799.

Lewis B, Waye J: Chronic gastrointestinal bleeding of obscure origin: The role of small bowel enteroscopy. *Gastroenterol* 1988;94:1117.

Tada M, Kawai K: Small bowel endoscopy *Scand J Gastroenterol* 1984;19:39.

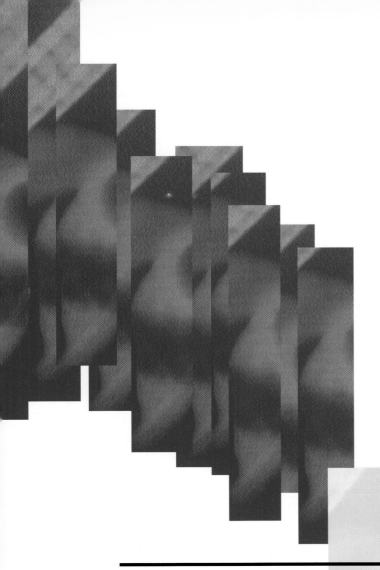

Endoscopic Sphincterotomy

Ramu P. Venu, MD
Joseph E. Geenen, MD

7

INTRODUCTION

The distal ends of the common bile duct and pancreatic duct traverse the duodenal wall before entering the intestine at the papilla of Vater—a smooth, nipple-like elevation located in the posteromedial wall of the descending duodenum. The intramural portion of the common bile duct varies in length from 2 to 8 mm. In over 80% of patients, the pancreatic duct and common bile duct merge into a common channel, the ampulla of Vater, before opening into the duodenum at the papilla. The intramural segments of the common bile duct and pancreatic duct are entwined by smooth muscle fibers which control the flow of bile and pancreatic secretions. This muscle, the sphincter of Oddi, is incised during endoscopic sphincterotomy (Fig. 7.1).

ENDOSCOPIC SPHINCTEROTOMY

Endoscopic sphincterotomy (ES) is a therapeutic modality that incises the papilla and sphincter muscles surrounding the distal common bile duct using electrodiathermy. This procedure, also known as papillotomy, was introduced in Germany and Japan in 1973, using slightly different techniques. Indications for ES have been growing steadily and now, with extensive experience, its role as a therapeutic alternative to operative management of patients with certain types of common bile duct obstruction has gained acceptance all over the world. It is the therapy of choice in patients with common bile duct stones and is successful in removing gallstones in 90% of such patients. ES has a relatively low complication rate and requires only a brief period of hospitalization.

INDICATIONS

Two major indications for ES are the management of patients with recurrent or residual common bile duct stones and papillary stenosis. Endoscopic sphincterotomy is especially useful in removing gallstones from the common bile duct in postcholecystectomy patients without a T-tube. In patients with an intact gallblad-

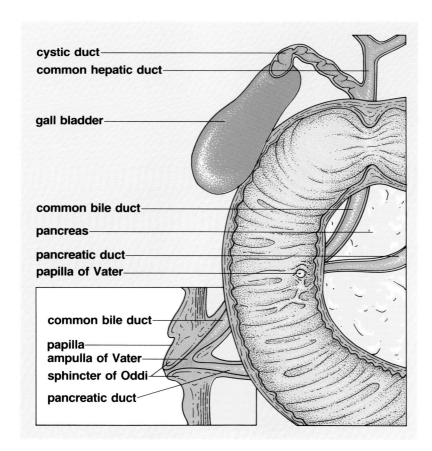

cystic duct
common hepatic duct

gall bladder

common bile duct
pancreas
pancreatic duct
papilla of Vater

common bile duct
papilla
ampulla of Vater
sphincter of Oddi
pancreatic duct

FIGURE 7.1 Anatomy of the common bile duct. The common hepatic duct joins the cystic duct to form the common bile duct which traverses through the head of the pancreas and empties into the duodenum through the ampulla of Vater. This intraduodenal portion of the common bile duct is enveloped by circular and longitudinal smooth muscle fibers forming the sphincter of Oddi. The papilla is usually located in the second portion of the duodenum in its posteromedial wall.

der who are at high operative risk, ES seems to be a reasonable alternative therapy for removing common bile duct stones. This technique also plays an important role in enlarging the papillary orifice as a preliminary step for the introduction of endoprosthesis, nasobiliary catheter, or Gruntzig balloon for dilatation of biliary strictures. Other indications for ES include sphincter of Oddi dysfunction, pancreatitis associated with gallstones and tumors of the papilla. ES may also be performed in sump syndrome which is a rare clinical entity encountered in patients who have had a side-to-side choledochoduodenostomy. Gallstones or food debris accumulated in the defunctionalized segment of the distal common bile duct may lead to biliary tract obstruction and ascending cholangitis in these patients. Following ES, the distal common bile duct can be cleared of such gallstones and debris. This technique is also indicated in unroofing a choledochocele which results from herniation or prolapse of the intramural segment of the common bile duct. A choledochocele may be associated with biliary colic, recurrent pancreatitis, or jaundice (Table 7.1).

More recently, ES has been utilized effectively to manage problems associated with laparoscopic cholecystectomy, such as retained common bile duct stones or bile duct injury with or without bile leak. Endoscopic sphincterotomy has also been occasionally performed to remove stone fragments from the common bile duct of patients who have had extracorporeal shock-wave lithotripsy for gallbladder stones.

Contraindications for ES are relatively few. Significant coagulation defects may pose a major risk of severe bleeding following ES. Similarly, in patients with long strictures of the distal common bile duct, ES may not be advisable. ES may be avoided if the endoscopist is uncertain of the anatomy of the sphincter area, especially when the sphincterotome cannot be positioned properly in the intramural segment of the common bile duct or Vaterian segment. In patients with very large common bile duct stones—larger than 25 mm in diameter—operative removal of gallstones may be preferred. Alternative, nonoperative therapies for these patients include the use of a lithotripter to crush gallstones, gallstone dissolution agents, and/or endoprostheses.

Peri-Vaterian diverticula, impacted gallstones at the ampulla with acute cholangitis or acute pancreatitis, or previous gastrectomy with a Billroth II anastomosis are not contraindications for ES.

EQUIPMENT

A superb roentgenography unit with fluoroscopic and radiographic capabilities and provisions for spot filming is an essential part of the equipment needed for ES. The radiographic table must be able to be tilted to Trendelenberg or upright positions. In addition, a lateral-viewing endoscope, cannulating catheter, sphincterotome with an electrodiathermy unit, and instruments for stone extraction such as a balloon catheter, basket, and lithotripter are also necessary when performing ES.

An insulated lateral-viewing endoscope with an external diameter of 11 mm is available through different manufacturing companies. A 2.8 mm instrument channel in this endoscope will accept cannulating catheters of 5F to 7F diameter, sphincterotomes, Dormia baskets, nasobiliary catheters and other accessories. The newer video endoscopes provide an opportunity for all participants to observe the procedure simultaneously.

Most sphincterotomes consist of a long Teflon catheter and a cautery wire. The wire traverses the

---

TABLE 7.1 INDICATIONS FOR ENDOSCOPIC SPHINCTEROTOMY

- Residual or recurrent common bile duct stones following cholecystectomy
- Common bile duct stones in high surgical risk patients with gallbladder *in situ*
- Sphincter of Oddi dysfunction
- Tumors of papilla
- Choledochocele
- Gallstone pancreatitis

- As a preliminary step for stent placement, nasobiliary catheter, or balloon dilatation
- Sump syndrome
- Common bile duct stone–bile duct injury with bile duct leak or stricture following laparoscopic cholecystectomy
- Stone fragments in patients who have had extracorporeal shock-wave lithotripsy

---

entire Teflon tube and is exposed for a variable length of 20 to 30 mm near the tip of the sphincterotome. By applying traction on the proximal end of the wire, the distal end of the catheter bends to assume a semilunar configuration (Fig. 7.2). When blended current is applied, a sequential incision of the tissues in contact with the wire takes place. The proximal end of the sphincterotome has an injection port for contrast instillation and a retractable handle. Four different types of sphincterotomes are currently available (Fig. 7.3):

- Traction or pull type.
- Soma or push type.
- Sphincterotome designed for patients who have had Billroth II surgery.
- Needle-knife sphincterotome.

Although these four types of sphincterotomes have their individual roles in ES, the traction type is the one that has the maximum clinical application. The traction type sphincterotome itself is available in four different forms. (Fig. 7.4):

- **Regular sphincterotome.** The cutting wire ends approximately 3 to 4 mm from the tip of the sphincterotome and the length of exposed wire might vary from 20 to 30 mm.
- **Precut sphincterotome.** The cutting wire extends to the very end of the Teflon tube.
- **Modified regular sphincterotome.** The cutting wire enters the catheter approximately 3 to 4 cm from the tapered tip of the Teflon tube, allowing a generous portion of the catheter to extend beyond the entrance of the wire. Because of this additional

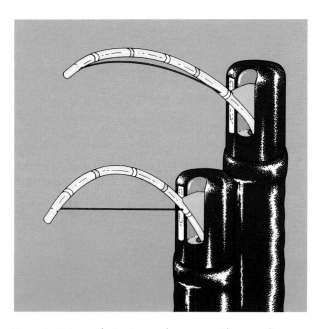

FIGURE 7.2 Lateral-viewing endoscopes with a regular sphincterotome protruding from the biopsy channel. The regular or pull-type sphincterotome assumes a characteristic bow shape when traction is applied on its proximal handle. This is the ideal position for incision during ES.

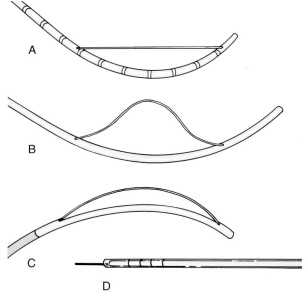

FIGURE 7.3 The most commonly used spincterotome, the traction or pull-type sphincterotome assumes a semilunar shape when the cutting wire is pulled taut **(A)**. In the Soma or push-type sphincterotome, the cutting wire protrudes outward when the handle is opened **(B)**. Note the distal portion of the sphincterotome itself is straight. The sphincterotome is designed for patients who have had Billroth II surgery. The cutting wire is directed in the opposite direction from that of the traction sphincterotome **(C)**. The needle-knife sphincterotome consists of a long wire with a 2 to 3 mm needle or knife at its tip **(D)**. This needle functions like a scalpel to incise the papilla.

length and the tapered tip, it is easier to cannulate the common bile duct in certain difficult cases. These features will also make it more likely that the sphincterotome is in the common bile duct and not the pancreatic duct. Also, this sphincterotome is less likely to slip out of the common bile duct when it is withdrawn for positioning the wire.

- **Guidewire sphincterotome.** This one has become popular in recent years, and can be slid over a guidewire that has already been placed in the bile duct. It is occasionally useful when free cannulation is difficult to achieve using conventional sphincterotomes. A guidewire is first passed in to the common bile duct through a cannula that has already been passed into the common bile duct. The cannula is then exchanged with the guidewire sphincterotome. There are two types of guidewire sphincteroromes:

- The **double-lumen sphincterotome** is provided with a lumen designed for the passage of the guidewire through its entire length (Fig 7.4D).
- The **single-lumen sphincterotome** has a small opening at its top to insert the guidewire. The outer diameter of these sphincterotomes vary from 5F to 7F.

The guidewire sphincterotomes come with a short or long tip, depending on the length of the polyethylene tube beyond the insertion of the cautery wire. When a

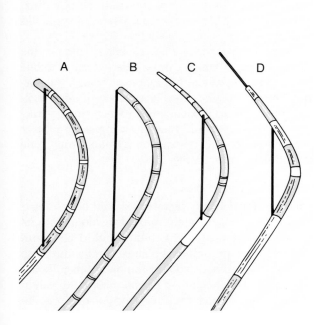

FIGURE 7.4 The traction-type sphincterotome is available in four different forms. The wire in a regular sphicterotome is inserted a few mm away from the tip (**A**). The wire in the precut sphincterotome extends up to the tip (**B**). With the modified regular sphincterotome, the cutting wire is inserted 3 cm away from the tip (**C**). Guidewire spinctero-tome is similar to traction-type sphincterotome with a lumen that allows the passage of a guidewire (**D**).

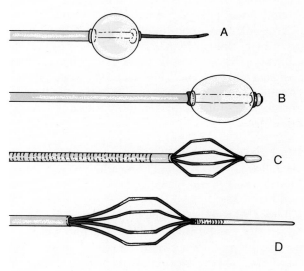

FIGURE 7.5 The double-lumen balloon catheter with a guidewire advanced through it (**A**). The balloon, located at the tip of the catheter, can be inflated with saline (**B**). The size of the inflated balloon varies from 8.5 to 15 mm in diameter and the catheter sizes vary from 5F to 7F. The four-wire basket with a helical shape is suitable for retrieving most stones (**C**). Some baskets are filiform with a flexible tip (**D**). This enables easy passage of the basket beyond large gallstones occluding the bile duct.

single-lumen spincterotome is used, the guidewire—0.18 to 0.35 inch—is passed through the opening at the tip of the sphincterotome and brought out through an artificially created hole just in front of the insertion of the cautery wire.

The direction of the cutting wire of the Soma sphincterotome is exactly opposite to the direction of the traction sphincterotome. With the wire opened up, the endoscopist pushes the Soma sphincterotome into the Vaterian segment such that the wire comes in contact with the tissues to be incised. Because of the difficulty in positioning the wire against the sphincter muscle, the Soma sphincterotome is less frequently used in the United States.

For patients who have had a Billroth II operation, two different types of sphincterotomes have been designed. The tip of both these sphincterotomes is straight, facilitating cannulation. One sphincterotome is sigmoid shaped, while the other one is similar to the Soma sphincterotome, which is straight at the distal end with the cutting wire emerging in the opposite direction.

The needle-knife sphincterotome consists of a Teflon catheter containing a long thin wire. A short 3 to 4 mm segment of this wire can be pushed out when traction is applied to the handle. Thus the needle-knife sphincterotome functions like a scalpel to incise the papilla when conventional sphincterotomy seems otherwise impossible.

STONE EXTRACTION EQUIPMENT

For gallstone retrieval, balloon catheters and stone extraction baskets are available.

Balloon Catheters. The balloon, located at the tip of the catheter, can be inflated with saline and will fluoroscopically produce a rounded, radiolucent shadow. A radiopaque ring located adjacent to the balloon enables localization of the catheter tip when the balloon is deflated. The size of the inflated balloon varies from 8.5 to 15 mm in diameter, and the catheter sizes are variable from 5F to 7F (Fig. 7.5B). There are two types of balloon catheters:

- A **two-lumen balloon catheter** allows injection of contrast through one of the lumens while the balloon is inflated with saline via the second lumen (Fig. 7.5A). Besides contrast instillation, the same lumen allows the passage of a guidewire for advancement of the catheter above the stone when it is otherwise difficult.

- A **single-lumen balloon** catheter will not permit the passage of a guidewire.

Stone Retrieval Baskets. Different styles of stone extraction baskets are also available varying in the orientation of wires and the size of the baskets. The size can vary from 22 to 30 mm in diameter and 30 to 70 mm in length. The four-wire baskets with a helical shape are suitable for retrieving most stones (Fig 7.5C). Smaller baskets may be especially useful for grasping and retrieving smaller stones. Baskets are also available with 3 to 8 wires. Some baskets are filiform with a flexible tip (Fig. 7.5D) that enables easy passage of the basket beyond large gallstones occluding the bile duct.

A mechanical lithotripter is used to crush stones and functions on the same principle as the stone extraction basket although its wires are stronger, thereby generating higher crushing pressures. To prevent stone/basket entrapment in the common bile duct, only baskets suitable for mechanical lithotripsy should be used for large stones greater than 1.5 cm.

Another accessory is a long nasobiliary catheter, the proximal end of which can be inserted into the bile duct and the distal end brought out through the nostril of the patient. Occasionally, it may be used to facilitate biliary drainage following ES when stone extraction is unsuccessful and there is an impending threat of common bile duct obstruction resulting from stone impaction (refer to Chapter 8).

PATIENT PREPARATION

The patient and family members should be informed in advance about the entire procedure along with its risks and complications. Patients should fast from midnight if the procedure is planned for the morning. Prophylactic antibiotic administration is generally not indicated unless the patient has an underlying valvular heart disease, biliary tract obstruction, or a pseudocyst of the pancreas. Coagulation studies consisting of prothrombin time, bleeding time, and platelet count should be done. In cases of coagulation abnormalities, necessary precautions should be taken to correct these using vitamin K injections, fresh frozen plasma, or administration of specific coagulation factors.

An intravenous line is started in the right arm and kept open using normal saline. Blood should be typed and stored for cross matching. Oropharyngeal anesthesia can be achieved by a local anesthetic. The patient is then placed in the supine position and a radiographic picture of the abdomen is taken. Such a radiograph is helpful to document any radiopaque shadow which might otherwise interfere with accurate interpretation of ductal anatomy. A radiopaque shadow may be caused by calcified vessels, calcification of the pancreas, or previously administered contrast material like barium. The patient is then turned to the recumbent prone position with both hands extended by his sides. Premedication is achieved by administering intravenous diazepam in doses of 10 to 20 mg, or midazolam (Versed) in doses of 2 to 10 mg. Opiates are generally avoided especially when sphincter of Oddi manometric studies are anticipated. These agents may cause sphincter spasm, making cannulation through the papilla difficult.

INTRODUCTION OF THE SPHINCTEROTOME

After adequate sedation, the endoscopist proceeds with intubation using a lateral-viewing endoscope and advancing it into the descending duodenum. Once there, the patient's position is readjusted so that the body is completely flat on the table. Glucagon, in doses of 0.2 mg, is administered intravenously to stop duodenal peristalsis. The glucagon might relax the sphincter muscle, facilitating cannulation. The papilla is identified and carefully observed for its location and size. A relatively large papilla might be a promising sign, as a reasonably long incision can be performed in such cases.

While a peripapillary diverticulum poses no contraindication for ES, extreme caution may be exercised to avoid duodenal perforation. In most instances, the papilla is located at the rim of a diverticulum although, rarely, it may be located between two diverticula (Fig. 7.6). Seldom is a papilla located inside a single diverticulum.

After localizing the papilla, the papillary orifice is identified and, using a cannula, a satisfactory cholangiogram is obtained. Though not absolutely necessary, a pancreatogram may be helpful. The cholangiogram is carefully reviewed for all its anatomical details, giving special attention to the intramural segment of the common bile duct or Vaterian segment (Fig. 7.7). A markedly dilated common bile duct and a long intramural segment will permit the endoscopist to perform an incision of 10 to 15 mm.

Next, the appropriate sphincterotome is selected. If a large stone is present in a dilated bile duct with a long intramural segment, a sphincterotome with a 30 mm exposed wire may be most suitable. With a small bile duct and a small papilla, as seen in patients with papillary stenosis, a sphincterotome with a 20 mm exposed wire may be less likely to cause perforation of the duodenal wall. Prior to inserting the sphincterotome into the scope, the endoscopist verifies the length of the flexed wire while the tip is taut by proximal manipulation by the GI assistant. A sphincterotome with a 30 mm exposed wire when taut will have a cutting length of 15 mm. However, as only half of the wire will be in contact with the tissue, a 7 mm incision during ES will be made.

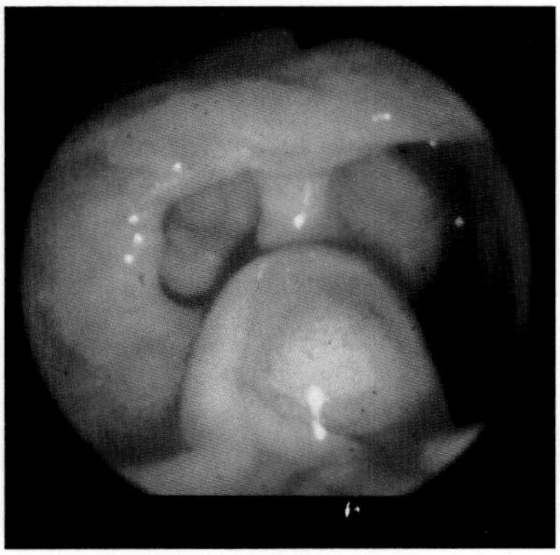

FIGURE 7.6 A papilla located between two diverticulum. The papilla is rather prominent in this case.

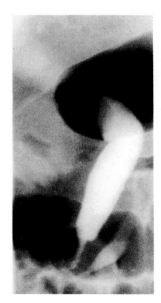

FIGURE 7.7 Cholangiogram of a patient with a long intramural segment of the common bile duct. Note that the intramural segment is characteristically narrow and tapering.

The sphincterotome is then introduced into the common bile duct. It might be helpful to position the endoscope very close to the papilla. If the sphincterotome cannot be advanced freely into the common bile duct, it is wedged at the superior margin of the papillary orifice at the 11 o'clock position. The elevator is partially closed and fixed in that position by pressing the thumb forcefully against the elevator control. The tip of the endoscope is then slowly withdrawn either by the endoscopist moving bodily away from the patient or by pulling back on the endoscope shaft with the right hand. Simultaneous manipulation of the vertical control will achieve the same effect in certain cases. This technique of impacting the sphincterotome at the superior margin and straightening the endoscope by withdrawing it slightly is the easiest and most common technique for advancing the sphincterotome into the bile duct when free cannulation cannot be achieved (Fig. 7.8).

If this technique fails, one might have to use the bowing technique. In this case the endoscope is positioned under the papilla and the superior margin of the papillary orifice is approached from a slight distance. Keeping the tip of the sphincterotome wedged at the superior margin, the same maneuvers as above can be repeated (Fig. 7.9). If these techniques fail, one may have to try a different traction type sphincterotome or change the patient's position partially to the left side.

SPHINCTEROTOMY TECHNIQUE

After cannulating the bile duct with the sphincterotome, the sphincterotome is advanced well inside the bile duct. The entire length of the exposed wire should be beyond the intramural segment. Its position in the common bile duct is reaffirmed by contrast instillation. The sphincterotome is then slowly withdrawn. As the wire becomes visible outside the papillary orifice, the GI assistant slowly tightens the wire to the partially flexed position by proximal manipulation of the sphincterotome (Fig. 7.10). The wire should be oriented to the 12 o'clock position of the papillary orifice to avoid injury to the duodenal wall or pancreatic duct (Fig. 7.11). When more than 50% of the wire is visible, a final radiographic picture is obtained and reviewed, thus ascertaining proper position of the sphincterotome (Fig. 7.12). Such a radiographic picture should indicate that:

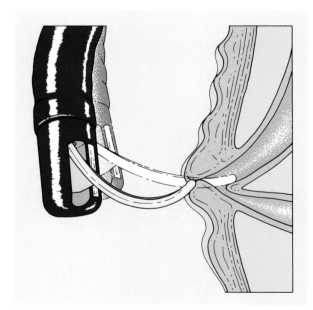

FIGURE 7.8 When the common bile duct cannot be freely cannulated, position the endoscope at some distance from the papilla and wedge the sphincterotome at the superior margin of the papillary orifice. Slowly pull back the endoscope, keeping the sphincterotome in place. This will often push the sphincterotome up into the common bile duct.

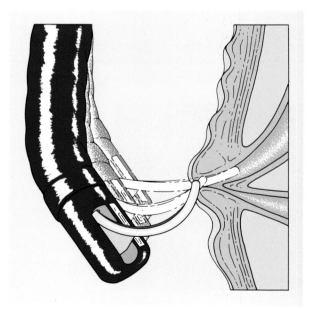

FIGURE 7.9 In the bowing technique, the endoscope is positioned under the papilla. By bowing the sphincterotome, the superior margin of the papillary orifice is approached from below in the attempt to push the sphincterotome into the common bile duct.

ENDOSCOPIC SPHINCTEROTOMY

- The sphincterotome is within the confines of the duodenal lumen and intramural segment of the common bile duct.
- It is oriented upward at a more or less acute angle to the long axis of the duodenal lumen.
- The wire of the sphincterotome is directed against the sphincter segment and is in the same plane as the Teflon catheter to which the wire is attached.

ELECTROCAUTERY INCISION

Accurate placement of the sphincterotome is the key to avoiding catastrophic complications from ES. Voice checks are made between the endoscopist and the GI assistant concerning the following preparations:

- Satisfactory application of the diathermy plate on the patient and its necessary connection.

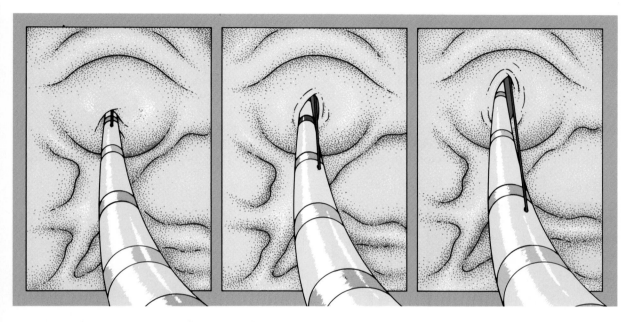

FIGURE 7.10 The sphincterotome is first inserted fully into the common bile duct. To remain within the intramural segment of the common bile duct, the sphincterotome is then slowly retracted into the duodenum. As the wire becomes visible outside the duct, it is gradually tightened to the partially flexed position. Approximately half of the wire should be visible outside the papillary orifice so only a portion of the papilla and the intramural segment of the common bile duct will be in contact with the cutting wire.

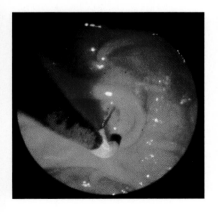

FIGURE 7.11 The papilla with the sphincterotome in position prior to ES. Note the wire is oriented to the 12 o'clock position of the papillary orifice to avoid injury to the duodenum or pancreatic duct.

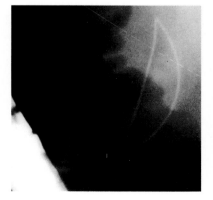

FIGURE 7.12 Radiograph of the distal common bile duct showing the sphincterotome in position. The wire, directed against the Vaterian segment, is in contact with the sphincter muscle.

- Attachment of the sphincterotome handle to the electrosurgical unit.
- Preparation of the electrosurgical unit with blended current setting—for example, 40 W when Valleylab diathermy unit is used.
- Appropriate orientation of foot switch pedal for easy use.
- Control of motility using glucagon.
- Degree of wire flexion required on the sphincterotome.
- Switching on the power just prior to cutting.

Before starting the electrocautery incision, the endoscope is slowly advanced 1 or 2 cm into the duodenum with simultaneous movement of the vertical control. This manipulation allows the endoscope to be positioned slightly away from the papilla, bringing the entire papilla and the intramural segment of the common bile duct under direct vision (Fig. 7.13). The endoscopist gently lifts the sphincterotome upward using the elevator, as blended current is applied in short bursts of 1 to 2 sec. Simultaneously, the endoscopist pulls up slowly on the sphincterotome. Current of 30 W to 50 W is used with the Valleylab model E3B cautery machine. This combination of movements will bring the cutting wire of the sphincterotome in contact with the tissues to be severed (Figs. 7.14). Only 3 to 7 mm of wire should be in contact with the papilla. Care must be taken to avoid pulling the sphincterotome out of the incised area as cutting proceeds. The endoscopist will be able to incise the tissue gradually from the papillary orifice to the transverse fold of the duodenum which forms a hood-like covering at the superior aspect of the papilla. Transected tissues include the papilla, the sphincter muscle and the intramural duct wall. (Fig. 7.15).

The length of the intramural segment of the common bile duct varies from patient to patient (Fig. 7.16). An approximate guide for the incision length can be made by observing the impression of the taut wire of

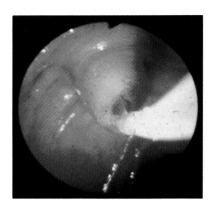

FIGURE 7.13 Sphincterotome advanced into the bile duct. The papilla, the transverse fold at its superior margin, and the surrounding duodenal mucosa are visible. The incision may be extended up to the transverse fold.

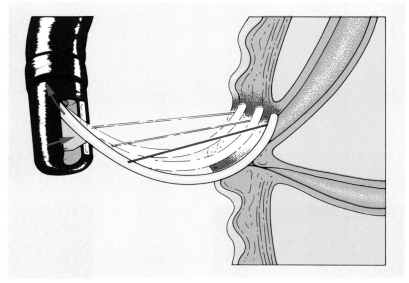

FIGURE 7.14 The sphincterotome is positioned in the Vaterian segment with the cutting wire pulled to the partially flexed position. Current is then applied in short bursts as the sphincterotome is pulled upward. As cutting proceeds, the wire may be kept in gentle contact with the tissue by raising it with the elevator and/or by pulling on the sphincterotome, as shown here. Care must be taken to avoid pulling the sphincterotome out of the incised area as cutting proceeds. Transected tissues include the papilla, the sphincter muscle and the intramural duct wall.

the sphincterotome on the intramural segment on the superior surface of the papilla and the duodenum. As a general rule, the incision is stopped when it reaches the transverse fold located superiorly to the papilla. If the papilla is small with a short intramural or Vaterian segment, the incisional length may be only 6 to 7 mm. However, in patients with a long Vaterian segment and dilated common bile duct, a generous incision of 15 to 20 mm can be made. A sphincterotome with a cutting wire of 30 mm will suffice to perform any incision from 6 to 20 mm.

A sudden gush of bile mixed with a small amount of bright red blood indicates complete incision of the sphincter choledochus. Fluoroscopically, one may visualize the entry of air from the duodenum into the biliary tree.

STONE EXTRACTION

Following ES, a deflated balloon catheter is advanced into the bile duct. Contrast material is instilled through the catheter to locate its position in the bile duct. When the tip of the catheter is above the stone to

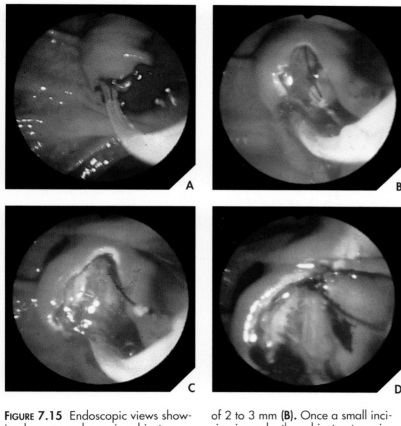

FIGURE 7.15 Endoscopic views showing how an endoscopic sphincterotomy incision is accomplished. The sphincterotome is positioned with half of the wire visible outside the papilla **(A)**. A small incision is made of 2 to 3 mm **(B)**. Once a small incision is made, the sphincterotome is repositioned and the incision is extended in increments of 2 to 3 mm **(C)**. Final view of completed incision. The papillary orifice is wide open **(D)**.

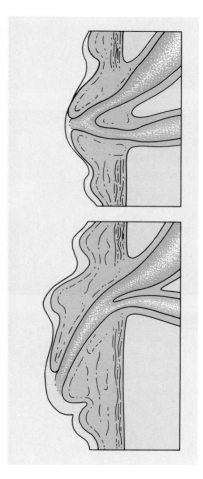

FIGURE 7.16 The length of the intramural segment of the common bile duct varies from patient to patient, ranging from a short 5 mm to a long 30 mm. The ES incision length is determined by the length of the intramural segment.

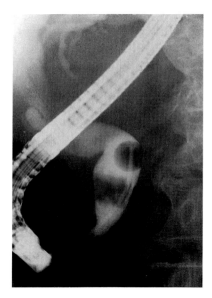

FIGURE 7.17 Radiographic picture showing stone extraction using balloon catheter. Note the fully inflated balloon located above the stone. The stone itself is seen as a square-shaped filling defect below the balloon. The bile duct is dilated.

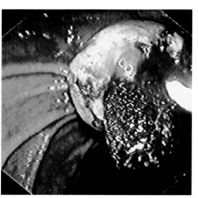 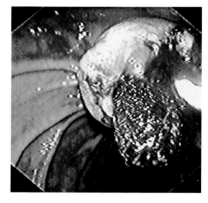

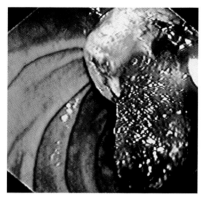 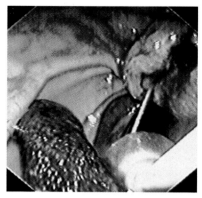

FIGURE 7.18 Endoscopic views depicting successful stone extraction using a balloon catheter. After an adequate ES, a balloon catheter is advanced into the bile duct above the gallstone. The balloon is inflated and as the balloon is pulled out through the papillary orifice, the stone slips out into the duodenum.

be extracted, the balloon is slowly inflated to 10 to 15 mm (Fig. 7.17). Keeping the balloon above the stone, the endoscopist pulls the catheter (Fig. 7.18). In most instances, the stone escapes through the enlarged papillary orifice followed by the balloon (Fig. 7.19).

Sometimes when a smaller stone is being extracted, it may slide alongside the balloon and migrate upward into the common hepatic duct or an intrahepatic duct. On the other hand, a light stone might float in relatively dense contrast medium and may be pushed further up into the intrahepatic duct by the force of contrast instillation. These undesirable situations can be avoided by raising the fluoroscopic table into the Trendelenburg position, which allows the stone to gravitate to the dependent distal bile duct thus making it more accessible for extraction. Occasionally it may be difficult to advance the balloon catheter above the stone. This problem is usually encountered when a stone is located proximally in a very tortuous bile duct.

Stacked multiple stones that fill the entire bile duct and stones wedged at the bifurcation are other instances where balloon catheter manipulation may be difficult. A double lumen balloon catheter can be extremely useful

under these circumstances. Initially, a guidewire is advanced alongside the stone until the wire tip is beyond the stone. The deflated balloon catheter is then slid over the guidewire. Once the balloon tip is above the stone, the guidewire may be removed, the balloon inflated, and the stone extracted (Fig. 7.20).

Generally, stones less than 12 mm in diameter can be extracted using a balloon catheter. Occasionally the stone may be wedged at the papillary orifice in the course of extraction. Sustained pressure, exerted by continuous pull on the catheter, may aid in stone extraction in such cases.

Stone extraction also can be performed using a Dormia basket. In this case, the basket with the wires closed is advanced into the bile duct above the stone. The basket is then opened and by gentle upward and downward movement, the stone is trapped within the basket (Fig. 7.21). Next the wire is tightened keeping the stone in a moderate grip inside the basket. The basket is pulled out of the duct into the duodenum. If the basket with the stone gets impacted at the papillary orifice, the endoscope may need to be pulled out of the patient by exerting some force, keeping a firm grip on the basket.

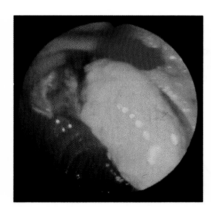

FIGURE 7.19 A stone, recently extracted during ES. lying in the duodenum.

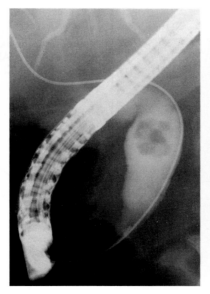

FIGURE 7.20 Initially, a guidewire is advanced alongside the stone until the wire tip is well beyond the stone. The deflated balloon catheter is then slid over the guidewire. Once the balloon tip is well above the stone, the balloon is inflated.

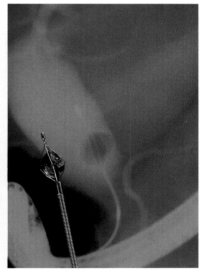

FIGURE 7.21 Radiograph taken during stone extraction using basket. In this case, the stone is trapped well inside the wire of the basket.

duct away from the papilla. The basket wire is connected to the cranking device and tightened. As the crank handle is turned, the wires are shortened, generating a crushing force against the entrapped stone.

Some lithotripters are not provided with a polyethylene sheath. Here cannulation is accomplished by the metal sheath, thus avoiding the additional step of exchanging the polyethylene catheter. When a 14F metal cable is used for crushing, the endoscope is removed and lithotripsy is done under fluoroscopic monitoring.

In a more recently available lithotripsy basket, a multisheath system is utilized. Here the basket wire containing the polyethylene sheath is covered with a metal sheath forming a second sleeve for the basket wire (Fig 7.24). When this new device is used, the bile duct is cannulated with the polyethylene catheter containing the basket. Next the basket is opened and the stone is entrapped. By proximal manipulation of the handle, the metal sheath is pushed over the catheter until it reaches the lower portion of the stone. Fragmentation is done by turning the handle on the cranking device.

This newer lithotripsy basket seems to offer the following advantages:

- It provides the catheter and metal sheath in a single unit, eliminating the need for exchanges.
- In patients with multiple stones, each stone can be fragmented, one after another, using the same basket without removing the basket.

ELECTROHYDRAULIC LITHOTRIPSY (EHL)

Electrohydraulic litrotripsy is another technique used to fragment stones. Electrohydraulic lithotripsy generates a spark in a water environment, producing a shock wave within the water. When the spark is generated very near the surface of the stone, the shock wave travels through the stone causing a fissure. With repeated shocks, this fissure will become deep and eventually the stone is fragmented. A newly available EHL probe has a built-in balloon catheter which, when inflated, forces the lithotripter tip to remain in the central axis of the duct, avoiding contact with the ductal wall (Fig 7.25).

EXTRACORPOREAL SHOCK-WAVE LITHOTRIPSY (ESWL)

Extracorporeal shock-wave lithotripsy has also been used for crushing large bile duct stones. The stone is targeted by fluoroscopy after injecting contrast material through a previously placed nasobiliary catheter or percutaneous catheter. Using ESWL, ducts have been cleared in approximately 80% of cases. Complications and the need for multiple lithotripsy sessions make this procedure somewhat less attractive.

LASER LITHOTRIPSY

In this modality, thermal energy generated by laser is utilized for stone fragmentation. Flash-lamp, pulsed

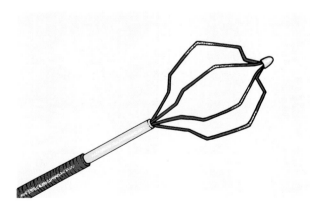

FIGURE 7.24 This basket wire containing a polyethylene sheath is covered with a metal sheath forming a second sleeve for the basket wire.

Neodynium-YAG laser has been found safe and effective in lithotripsy, both in laboratory animals and in human studies. The laser beam is carried to the stone via a percutaneous choledochoscope, mother-and-baby dual endoscope system and more recently using a specialized balloon basket or three-layer sleeve system. In the latter, the laser fiber is kept inside a 4F catheter that is advanced through a 10F polyethylene sleeve inserted into the bile duct; the stone is then targeted and laser beam applied. Laser lithotripsy has been useful in fragmentation in approximately 80% of cases attempted.

Balloon-tipped catheters have been used to focus the shock wave on the stone to avoid bile duct injury. Experience with this technique has shown some promising results.

CONTACT DISSOLUTION

Complete or partial dissolution of a common bile duct stone can be accomplished by continuous infusion of mono-octanoin through a previously placed nasobiliary catheter. The catheter tip should be above the stone. Infusion rate is kept at 2 to 5 cc/hr for 2 to 5 days. The effect of dissolution therapy can be checked by cholangiographic studies every 24 to 48 hrs. Mono-octanoin has been useful in partial or complete dissolution of common bile duct stones in approximately 50% of cases.

Methyl-tert-butyl-ether (MTBE) is another agent shown to be useful in dissolving cholesterol stones. Although no major untoward effects have been reported with MTBE, controlled infusion using a specialized pump system may be desirable for infusion. Experience with common bile duct stone is limited while its role in gallbladder stone dissolution by continuous infusion has been very promising.

If all attempts to remove stones fail, then an endoprosthesis can be inserted to facilitate biliary drainage and keep the stone from impacting and causing biliary obstruction (Fig. 7.26).

PATIENTS WITH BILLROTH II GASTRECTOMY

Endoscopic access to the papilla of Vater and its subsequent cannulation and ES can be difficult in patients who have had partial gastrectomies and Billroth II gastrojejunostomies. Quite often, the endoscopist may have to try different types of sphincterotomes to accomplish sphincterotomy.

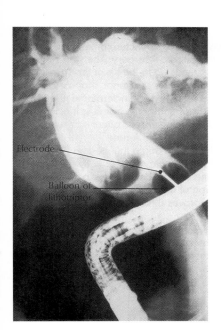

FIGURE 7.25 A newly available EHL probe has a built-in balloon catheter which, when inflated, allows the lithotripter tip to remain in the central axis of the duct.

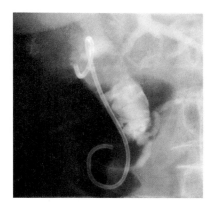

FIGURE 7.26 The common bile duct stone in this patient was large and difficult to extract. An endoprosthesis was placed to facilitate biliary drainage and to prevent stone impaction. The large stone can be seen in the distal portion of the bile duct.

ter muscle may then be incised using diathermy current (Fig. 7.31)

The Soehendra Billroth II sphincterotome may also be used when performing ES in certain patients. Once the bile duct is cannulated, the cutting wire is pushed out against the sphincter muscle. A radiographic picture must be taken to ensure proper orientation of the wire before incision is initiated (Fig 7.32). When current is applied, the reverse cutting wire produces an incision in a caudad direction as viewed endoscopically. As in the case of a needle-knife sphincterotomy, this results in a cephalad incision in relation to the actual anatomy of the papilla and common bile duct (Fig. 7.33) The sigmoid-shaped sphincterotome is rarely used now.

In general, ES in patients with partial gastrectomies and Billroth II anastomoses seems to be more difficult.

PATIENTS WITH DUODENAL DIVERTICULA
Extreme caution should be exercised in performing ES in patients with peripapillary diverticula. When the papilla is located at the rim of a diverticulum, the wire of the sphincterotome should be directed away from the diverticulum (Fig. 7.34). In situations where the papilla is located at the bottom of the diverticulum, incision lengths should be limited to the superior margin of the papilla. The key factors to consider to avoid complications are the direction of the sphincterotomy and the short incision length.

FOLLOW-UP
Following ES, the patient is observed for an hour in the recovery room. Pulse, respirations, and blood pressures are carefully monitored. Any abdominal discomfort, nausea, or vomiting is attended to when needed. If the vital signs are stable, the patient is then kept at complete bedrest for the next 6 to 8 hrs. A liquid diet can be given at this time. It is our practice to keep the patient in the hospital for the next 48 hrs. The intravenous line may be discontinued 24 hrs after the procedure, provided the patient remains in stable condition. The patient is carefully observed for any evidence of upper GI bleeding, pancreatitis, cholangitis, or other complications while in the hospital. At the time of discharge, the patient is instructed about the possibility of delayed GI bleeding and mild abdominal discomfort which may last for 1 to 2 weeks. If the stone extraction is successful and the incision remains wide open, no follow-up examination is necessary (Fig. 7.35). However, in patients who had papillary stenosis, follow-up examination may be necessary since the incidence of restenosis is high for this group. This may be carried out at 3 months, 1 year, or when the symptoms return.

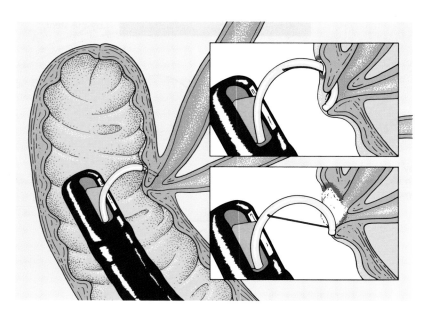

FIGURE 7.31 Another approach for patients who have had Billroth II gastrectomies is using the needle-knife sphincterotome. This sphincterotome is placed between the papillary orifice and the transverse fold. When current flow is initiated, the knife burrows through the papillary wall to reach the ampulla, thus creating a choledochoduodenal fistula. A traction type sphincterotome is then introduced through this opening and gently advanced until it exits through the papillary orifice. The intervening sphincter muscle is then incised.

RESOLUTION OF UNUSUAL PROBLEMS

The ability to advance a spincterotome selectively and repeatedly into the bile duct and to orient the wire properly form the basis for successful ES. Occasionally, the papilla may be too small or the Vaterian anatomy so altered that the endoscopist will find it difficult to advance the sphincterotome more than a few millimeters. Contrast instillation under these circumstances may opacify the bile duct to identify a stone.

When free cannulation of the common bile duct cannot be accomplished, ES becomes a difficult procedure. Some other techniques successfully employed in such instances are:

• Guidewire sphincterotomy.
• Needle-knife sphincterotomy.
• Sphincterotomy using a precut sphincterotome.

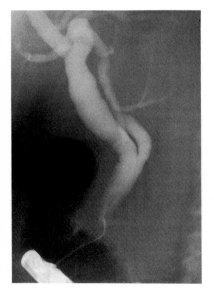

FIGURE 7.32 This radiographic image from a Billroth II patient shows the cutting wire of the Soehendra–type sphincterotome pushed out against the sphincter muscle proper. This image ensures proper orientation before incision.

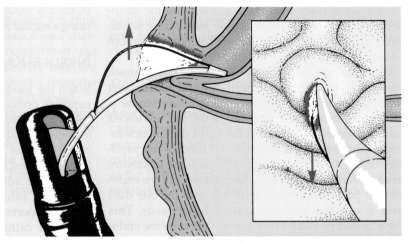

FIGURE 7.33 Note the Billroth II sphincterotome being used to perform ES. The cutting wire is pushed out instead of being flexed in a bow position.

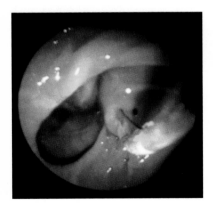

FIGURE 7.34 A patient with duodenal diverticulum. The papilla is located at the rim of the diverticulum. The wire of the sphincterotome, which is partially open, is oriented away from the diverticulum to avoid perforation.

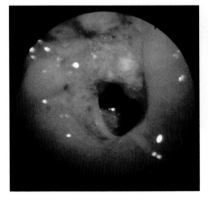

FIGURE 7.35 Appearance of papillary orifice 3 months postprocedure. The incision has completely healed. Note the papillary orifice is wide open.

cautery is activated. The papillary orifice is slightly enlarged and the wire may be tightened more to bring it into contact with the superior margin of the incision to complete the sphincterotomy. Of all ES techniques, this is the least commonly employed since it may be associated with an increased incidence of complications.

RELATED COMPLICATIONS

Following ES, the patient should be closely observed for any immediate or delayed complications. A survey conducted by the American Society for Gastrointestinal Endoscopy indicates a complication rate of 6.7% associated with ES (Table 7.2). Major complications noted in this study include bleeding, perforation, pancreatitis, cholangitis and trapped baskets. The mortality rate was 0.4%.

Bleeding from the sphincterotomy site constitutes the most common complication. The vast majority of bleeding occurs immediately following the procedure. Massive bleeding almost always results when the retroduodenal artery is severed. Fortunately, this crucial vessel is located away from the papillary orifice in all but 5% of patients, where it may course through the dangerous zone.

There are several therapeutic options available to control bleeding. Tamponade using an inflated balloon catheter should be attempted first. Local instillation of epinephrine 1:10,000 (5 to 10 mL), 98% ethanol (1 to 2 mL), or sodium morrhuate (3 to 5 mL) using a sclerotherapy needle 5 mm long has been tried with variable success. Cauterization using heater probe or bipolar electrode may occasionally be useful. If bleeding continues in spite of these therapeutic measures, arterial embolization or operative intervention should be considered. Rarely bleeding may take place 2 or 3 days following ES. Most of these bleeding episodes stop spontaneously; however, the patient should be cautioned about this complication at the time of discharge and instructed not to take any antiplatelet drugs, including aspirin, for several days.

Acute pancreatitis is another serious complication. Severe abdominal pain, nausea, vomiting, signs of ileus with abdominal distention and absent bowel sounds, fever, leukocytosis, and elevated amylase are the typical signs and symptoms seen in patients with postsphincterotomy pancreatitis. The majority of patients with pancreatitis respond well to medical treatment—nasogastric suction and IV fluids.

The incidence of pancreatitis can be reduced by careful cannulation of the common bile duct. Cannulation of the pancreatic duct repeatedly with the sphincterotome should be avoided by all means. Orientation of the electrocautery wire should be between the 11 and 1 o'clock position of the papillary orifice and not toward the 3 o'clock position. The amount of coagulation current used at ES should be minimal.

Another significant complication associated with ES is duodenal perforation. The patient usually com-

---

TABLE 7.2 ENDOSCOPIC SPHINCTEROTOMY COMPLICATIONS

Total patients in whom endoscopic sphincterotomy was attempted = 5790

	NO. OF PATIENTS	SURGERY REQUIRED	DEATHS
Bleeding (nontransfused)	38	0	0
Bleeding (transfused)	85	18	11
Pancreatitis	122	5	6
Perforation	57	28	1
Cholangitis	78	26	2
Trapped basket	13	9	2
Total	393 (6.8%)	86 (22%)*	22 (0.37%)

*22% of 393 patients who had complications
Reproduced from Tedesco FJ, Vennes JA Dreyer M: In: Okabe H, Honda T, Oshiba F, eds. *Endoscopic Surgery* New York, NY:Elsevier;1984:41.

plains of severe abdominal pain and a flat plate roentgenogram of the abdomen usually shows air outside the confinement of the duodenum in the retroperitoneal area. Acute pancreatitis and retroduodenal perforation may be difficult to differentiate from one another. Just like pancreatitis, most duodenal perforations can be managed medically by nasogastric suction, IV fluids and broad spectrum antibiotics. Duodenal perforation may be complicated by retroperitoneal abscess formation. Serial CT scan examination is important in identifying this serious complication as operative drainage is then indicated.

Duodenal perforation most commonly occurs in patients with a small papilla, short intramural segment, a nondilated common bile duct, or papillary stenosis. Duodenal perforation clearly results from an incision which is longer than the intramural segment of the common bile duct. Using a short wire length during electrocautery incision and keeping at least half of the wire outside the papillary orifice is the key to avoid this serious complication.

Trapped basket is another rare complication. The basket containing a large stone becomes wedged at the papillary orifice and cannot be pulled out of the bile duct. In this situation the basket wire is disconnected from the handle, and the endoscope is withdrawn over the basket. The catheter is then exhanged with a metal sheath or cable which under fluoroscopic monitoring, is advanced into the duodenum up to the papilla. The basket wire is then connected to a cranking

device and mechanical lithotripsy may be attempted by turning the handle on the cranking device. Following lithotripsy, the basket can be removed with the crushed stones.

Another option is to enlarge the sphincterotomy incision. A needle-knife sphincterotome or a traction sphincterotome (Fig. 7.40) may be advanced through the endoscope. The sphincterotome is placed at the superior margin of the previous incision which is then extended by 3 to 4 mm. The basket subsequently may be pulled out. Occasionally, the basket may escape spontaneously from the common bile duct into the duodenum. Rarely a basket may have to be removed by operative intervention.

Ascending cholangitis resulting from impaction of the stone at the edematous papilla is another complication. In this instance, the stone may be dislodged using an inflated balloon of a balloon catheter. If stone removal is unsuccessful, a nasobiliary catheter is passed above the stone and drainage is established to prevent future episodes of stone impaction. Appropriate antibiotic therapy may then be initiated. Cholangitis can be prevented in most instances if gallstones are extracted during ES.

CONCLUSIONS

The incidence of complications associated with ES may be decreased by adhering to certain technical details. Patients should stop taking aspirin or similar

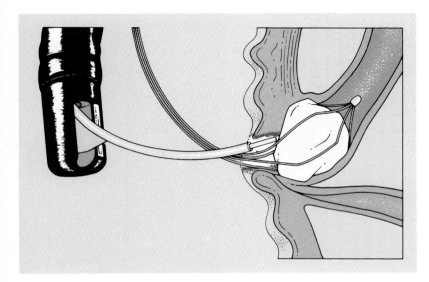

FIGURE 7.40 When a basket containing a large stone is trapped at the papillary orifice, the basket handle is severed and the endoscope is pulled out over the basket catheter. Using a needle-knife sphincterotome, the incision may be enlarged so that the basket can be retrieved. It may also fall out spontaneously.

antiplatelet agents or anticoagulants a week to 10 days prior to ES. Coagulation studies should be obtained prior to ES and any abnormality encountered should be corrected. Blood should be available for immediate transfusion. In general, the longer the incision length, the higher the chance for bleeding from the incision. Therefore, the incision length should be controlled by cutting at increments of 2 to 3 mm at a time. Blended current may be preferable to cutting current for incision. In the presence of overt bleeding, subsequent instrument management such as use of balloon catheter or basket may be avoided until the bleeding is controlled.

REFERENCES

Bedogni G, Bertoni G, Contini S, et al: Endoscopic sphincterotomy in patients with Billroth II partial gastrectomy. Comparison of three different techniques. *Gastrointest Endosc* 1984;30:300.

Classen M, Safrany L: Endoscopic papillotomy and removal of gallstones. *Br Med J* 1975;4:371.

Cotton PB, Chapman M, Whiteside CG, LeQuesne LP: Duodenoscopic papillotomy and gallstone removal. *Br J Surg* 1976;63:709.

Cotton PB, Vallon AG: British experience with duodenoscopic sphincterotomy for removal of bile duct stones. *Br J Surg* 1981;68:373.

Cotton PB, Kozarek RA, Schapiro RH, et al: Endoscopic laser lithotripsy of large bile duct stones. *Gastroenterology* 1990;99:1128.

Cotton PB, Lehman G, Vennes J, et al: Endoscopic sphincterotomy complications and their management. An attempt at consensus. *Gastrointest Endosc* 1991;37:383.

Geenen JE, Hogan WJ, Shaffer, RD, Stewart ET, Dodds WJ, Arndorfer RC: Endoscopic electrosurgical papillotomy and manometry in biliary tract disease. *JAMA* 1977;237:2075.

Geenen JE, Vennes JA, Silvis SE: Resume of a seminar on endoscopic retrograde sphincterotomy (ERS). *Gastrointest Endosc* 1981;27:31.

Huibregtse K, Katon R, Tytgat GNJ: Precut papillotomy via fine needle knife papillotome: A safe and effective technique. *Gastrointest Endosc* 1986;32:403.

Katon RM, Bilbao MK, Parent JA, Smith FW: Endoscopic retrograde cholangiopancreatography in patients with gastrectomy and gastrojejunostomy (Billroth II): A case for the forward look. *Gastrointest Endosc* 1975;21:164.

Lux G: Endoscopic papillotomy: the development of a method. *Endoscopy* 1978;10:206.

Osnes M, Myren J: Endoscopic retrograde cholangiopancreatography (ERCP) in patients with Billroth II partial gastrectomies. *Endoscopy* 1975;15:227.

Reiter JJ, Bayer HP, Mennicken L et al: Results of endoscopic papillotomy: a collective experience from nine endoscopic centers in West Germany. *World J Surg* 1978;2:505.

Sackmann M, Delius M, Sauerbruch T, et al: Shock-wave lithotripsy of gallbladder stones. The first 175 patients. *N Engl J Med* 1988;318:393.

Safrany L: Duodenoscopic sphincterotomy and gallstone removal. *Gastroenterol* 1977;72:37.

Safrany L: Endoscopy and retrograde cholangiopancreatography after Billroth II operation. *Endoscopy* 1982; 4:198.

Seifert F: Endoscopic papillotomy and removal of gallstones. *Am J Gastroenterol* 1978;69:154.

Siegel JH: Endoscopic management of choledocholithiasis and papillary stenosis. *Surg Gynecol Obstet* 1979; 148:747.

Stout DJ, Sivak MV, Sullivan BH: Endoscopic sphincterotomy and removal of gallstones. *Surg Gynecol Obstet* 1980;150:673.

Tedesco FJ, Vennes JA, Dreyer M: Endoscopic sphincterotomy: The USA experience in endoscopic surgery. In: Okabe H, Honda T, Oshiba F, eds: *Endoscopic Surgery* New York,NY: Elsevier; 1984:41.

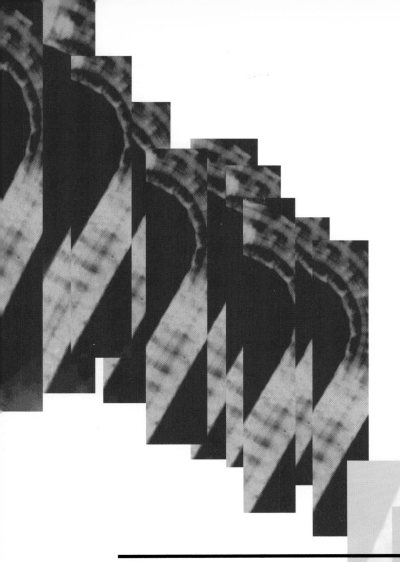

Endoscopic Management of Biliary Tract Obstruction

Joseph E. Geenen, MD
Rama P. Venu, MD

8

INTRODUCTION

A variety of clinical disorders leading to biliary tract obstruction can be effectively managed by endoscopic therapy. Endoscopic sphincterotomy (ES), the forerunner of such therapeutic modalities, has been shown to be successful in 90% of patients with common bile duct stones (refer to Chapter 7). New endoscopic procedures, including placement of a nasobiliary catheter (NBC) or endoprosthesis, and balloon dilatation of biliary strictures, have been developed for the management of noncalculous causes of biliary tract obstruction. These innovative measures for biliary drainage are very encouraging, since they compare favorably with operative biliary bypass in morbidity and mortality rates while avoiding general anesthesia and prolonged hospitalization.

The techniques used in performing these procedures have evolved as an extension of endoscopic retrograde cholangiopancreatography (ERCP) and ES. Therefore, the endoscopist should have extensive prior experience performing ERCP and ES before attempting these new therapeutic techniques in the biliary tree (Fig. 8.1).

NASOBILIARY CATHETER (NBC)

Temporary or short-term biliary decompression can be accomplished by placing an NBC above common bile duct stones or strictures in the biliary tract. An NBC consists of a long polyethylene tube, one end of which is placed inside the biliary tree while the other end exits through the nostril and connects to a bile drainage bag. The NBC can thus function like a T-tube.

INDICATIONS

There are a number of indications for NBC placement (Table 8.1). The most common is unsuccessful stone extraction following ES. In this situation, there is the potential danger of biliary tract obstruction secondary to impaction of gallstones at the papillary orifice. NBC can prevent such stone impaction and establish biliary drainage while an assessment is made of the feasibility of later extending the sphincterotomy incision length.

An NBC in this situation also provides access for a second option of perfusing the common bile duct for 5 to 10 days with monooctanoin, a gallstone-dissolving agent with a 50% success rate. Monooctanoin is con-

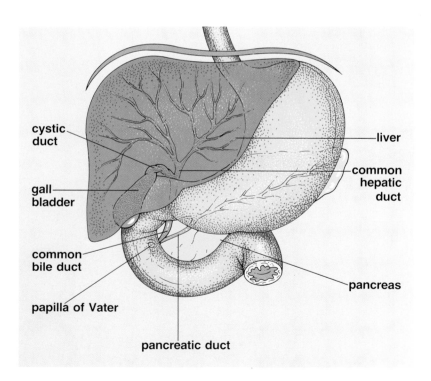

FIGURE 8.1 Anatomy of the biliary tree. The right and left intrahepatic ducts form the common hepatic duct at the porta hepatis. The cystic duct may join the common hepatic duct close to the ampulla or as high as the proximal hepatic duct. Below the entry point of the cystic duct is the common bile duct which joins the pancreatic duct before their final duodenal exit at the papilla of Vater.

cystic duct

gall bladder

common bile duct

papilla of Vater

pancreatic duct

liver

common hepatic duct

pancreas

tinuously pumped into the bile duct at the rate of 2 to 7 mL/hr through an NBC, the tip of which should be above the gallstone. After establishing a suitable rate of infusion which the patient can tolerate without severe abdominal pain or diarrhea, the infusion can be continued on an outpatient basis. Alternately, 3 to 10 mL/hr of monooctanoin can be administered every hour using a syringe, after removal of a similar amount of bile from the bile duct. The indwelling NBC also allows periodic cholangiograms to evaluate the stone size to assess the effectiveness of monooctanoin treatment.

Methyl-tert-butyl-ether (MTBE) is another pharmacological agent used for contact dissolution. MTBE can be delivered through a modified nasobiliary catheter and slowly infused with the aid of a specialized infusion pump.

Nasobiliary catheters have also been used to infuse antibiotics in cases of severe acute bacterial cholangitis. In patients with sclerosing cholangitis, multiple strictures and segmental dilatation of the biliary tract is characteristically seen on cholangiographic studies. The intrahepatic ducts may contain small stones or biliary sludge. Using an NBC, continuous perfusion of the biliary tree with normal saline,—1,000 mL/24 hr, —might flush the intrahepatic biliary tree of sludge or small stones, and corticosteroid infusion may decrease the chronic inflammatory reaction leading to intrahepatic obstruction.

The presence of jaundice increases the morbidity and mortality in patients undergoing elective biliary tract surgery. In these patients with extrahepatic biliary tract obstruction, an NBC can decrease the jaundice, providing preoperative biliary decompression, which may decrease the perioperative complications.

In the patient who is septic or has severe coagulopathy, an NBC can be temporarily positioned in the biliary tree to decompress a tight stricture without performing ES. This can be done with relative ease and with little or no risk. Once the infection has been controlled or the coagulopathy corrected, ES can be performed on an elective basis and a large endoprosthesis inserted for long-term therapy.

An NBC may also provide access for intraluminal irradiation therapy using iridium.

Another emerging indication of NBC is for the management of common bile duct stones using extracorporeal shock-wave lithotripsy (ESWL). Cholangiogram through NBC is necessary to outline the common bile duct stone and for targeting stone for delivery of shock waves during ESWL.

Equipment

Equipment needed for nasobiliary catheter placement includes an NBC with connecting bag and washer, guidewires of different sizes, a short nasopharyngeal or nasogastric tube, and grasping forceps.

Nasobiliary catheters are available in two sizes, 5F and 7F, both of which can be advanced through the 2.8 mm instrument channel of a lateral-viewing endoscope with an external diameter of 11 mm. The tip of the NBC placed in the bile duct has several side holes

---

TABLE 8.1 INDICATIONS FOR NASOBILIARY CATHETERS

Biliary decompression	Biliary perfusion	Miscellaneous
• Ascending cholangitis secondary to impaction of stone • Ascending cholangitis in patients with stones in the common bile duct and coagulopathy • Preoperative biliary decompression to decrease severe jaundice secondary to extrahepatic biliary obstruction	• Gallstone dissolution agents, such as monooctanoin • Antibiotics in patients with ascending cholangitis • Corticosteroids in patients with sclerosing cholangitis	• Intraluminal radiation therapy in selected cases of malignant stricture • For targeting common bile duct stones during extracorporeal shock-wave lithotripsy

---

to facilitate adequate bile flow. To prevent catheter dislodgment, earlier models of NBCs had a pigtail-shaped curl at the end, whereas the newest type has a straight end with an alpha-shaped curl in the duodenal portion to maintain its position (Fig. 8.2).

The standard guidewire is 400 cm long and 0.035 inches in diameter. The tip of the guidewire that negotiates the bile duct is blunt and flexible. Small-caliber guidewires are also available, with diameters of 0.018 in to 0.025 in.

Specially designed nasopharyngeal tubes are available for transposing NBCs through the nostrils. They are 25 cm long and 16F in diameter. The tip that is inserted through the nostril is rounded and smooth, but, unlike a standard nasogastric tube, there are no side holes in a nasopharyngeal tube. If a special nasopharyngeal tube is not available, a 16F Levine tube or nasogastric tube of any kind may be shortened to 25 to 30 cm and used for this purpose.

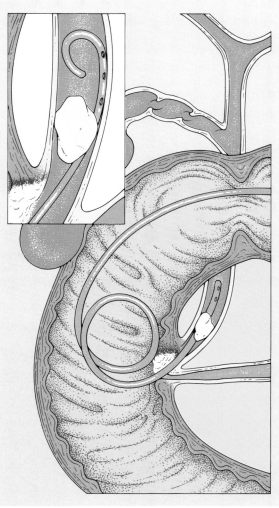

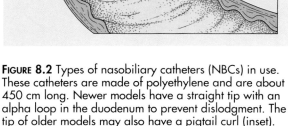

FIGURE 8.2 Types of nasobiliary catheters (NBCs) in use. These catheters are made of polyethylene and are about 450 cm long. Newer models have a straight tip with an alpha loop in the duodenum to prevent dislodgment. The tip of older models may also have a pigtail curl (inset).

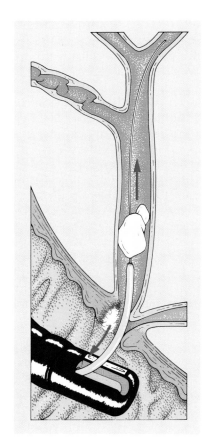

FIGURE 8.3 The cannula containing the guidewire is advanced into the common hepatic duct at its bifurcation. The cannula is withdrawn in 1 cm to 2 cm increments as the guidewire is advanced into the common bile duct. These synchronous movements in opposite directions keep the guidewire position stationary at the bifurcation of the common hepatic duct.

Nasobiliary Catheter Placement Technique

An endoscopic sphincterotomy is usually performed prior to NBC placement with the notable exception of a patient with fulminant cholangitis or a severe coagulopathy complicating biliary tract obstruction. Nasobiliary catheter placement can be performed in the following steps:

- Cannulation of the common bile duct with a 5F or 7F cannula.
- Advancement of the guidewire through the cannula.
- Withdrawal of the cannula over the guidewire.
- Advancement of the NBC over the guidewire into the bile duct after the guidewire is cleaned and sprayed with silicone.
- Withdrawal of the endoscope over the NBC.
- Transposition of the NBC through the nose.
- Taping of the NBC to the cheek and connecting it to a drainage bag.

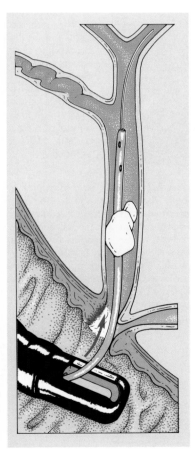

FIGURE 8.4 The guidewire is advanced all the way into the common hepatic duct, well above the stones. The NBC then enters the ampulla through the incised papillary orifice over the guidewire. Care is taken to avoid loop formation and the endoscope is placed close to the papilla.

Before positioning the NBC in the biliary tree, the endoscopist should review the cholangiogram to be familiar with the anatomy of the biliary tract, assessing the length and location of the stricture or the size and number of stones.

The same cannula used for cannulating the bile duct during ERCP is carefully advanced well up the biliary tree. The cannula should be above the level of the stricture or stones. Contrast medium, 2 to 5 mL, is instilled through the cannula to locate the tip of the cannula. The cannula is then cleared of the contrast by injection of 5 to 10 mL of normal saline, ensuring that contrast material will not adhere to the inner surface of the cannula and cause difficulty in advancing the guidewire.

An appropriate guidewire of 400 cm for exchange is selected. The flexible or floppy end of the guidewire is placed through the cannula and slowly advanced into the bile duct. The guidewire should be kept straight, which is most easily achieved by having the GI assistant stand at a distance, and hold the straight guidewire end taut. The endoscope's position should be close to the papilla, preferably inferior to and looking upward toward it. Keeping the papilla in view, the endoscopist makes tip adjustments as needed to maintain the desired entry angle while simultaneously observing the guidewire advancement fluoroscopically. Communication between the endoscopist and the GI assistant is helpful in coordinating each step of the procedure.

Once the guidewire has been properly sited well inside the hepatic duct, the cannula is slowly removed over the long guidewire. To maintain the guidewire's position above the stricture or stone, the endoscopist withdraws the cannulating catheter as the GI assistant advances the guidewire (Fig. 8.3). Fluoroscopy is used intermittently to verify the guidewire position.

The external portion of the guidewire is cleaned with water and sprayed with silicone. An appropriate NBC is selected. The tapered or curved end of the NBC is threaded over the guidewire and slowly advanced through the instrument channel of the endoscope. As the NBC exits from the endoscope, the elevator is opened so that the catheter tip will not impact onto the elevator mechanism. By gently pushing, the NBC advances steadily over the guidewire into the bile duct (Fig. 8.4). The endoscopist must constantly watch the duodenum and ampulla to prevent loop formation of either the NBC or the guidewire inside the duodenum. Fluoroscopic monitoring is continued while the NBC is advanced and the GI assistant keeps the guidewire taut. Once the NBC reaches the desired position above the obstruction in the bile duct, the guidewire is removed.

The endoscope is slowly withdrawn over the NBC. Again, this is accomplished by a coordinated team effort by the endoscopist, radiology technician, and GI assistant. By intermittent fluoroscopic observation, the radiology technician confirms that the tip of the NBC is not displaced. While the endoscopist advances the NBC, the GI assistant withdraws the endoscope in increments of 1 or 2 cm. This maintains the stationary position of the NBC. After the endoscope and mouth guard are removed from the patient, the entire catheter position is viewed fluoroscopically (Fig. 8.5). Loops or extra length in the NBC in the throat, esophagus, stomach, or duodenum are undesirable and are straightened or removed by gently pulling on the NBC. Ideally, the end of the pigtail or straight tip catheter should be well above the obstruction or stone. There should be a loop in the descending portion of

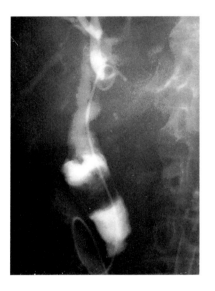

FIGURE 8.5 Radiograph showing an NBC in the bile duct of a patient with two retained common bile duct stones. In this case, the pigtail loop of the NBC is located above the bigger stone.

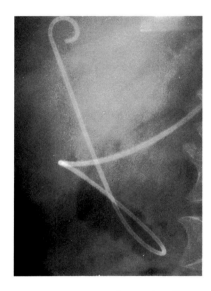

FIGURE 8.6 NBC after placement in the bile duct. The pigtail curl is most likely in the intrahepatic duct, but is not visible because the contrast medium has drained out. The small loop in the descending duodenum prevents displacement. The remainder of the NBC is coursing through the duodenal bulb, pylorus, and stomach.

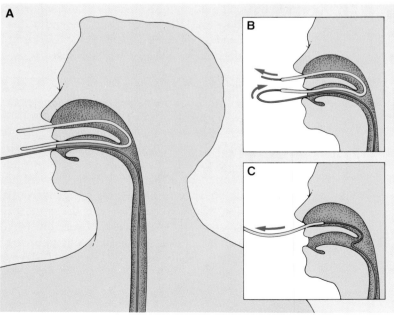

FIGURE 8.7 The NBC exits through the mouth. A nasopharyngeal tube has been advanced through the nose and brought out through the mouth (**A**). The NBC is then threaded through the oral end of the nasopharyngeal catheter until it passes out through the nasal end of the nasopharyngeal tube (**B**). Slow pulling on the nasopharyngeal tube will bring the NBC out through the nose (**C**).

the duodenum to prevent migration. This can be created by curling a portion of the NBC under fluoroscopic monitoring. The remaining section of the NBC through the stomach and the esophagus should be straight (Fig. 8.6).

Although the NBC now emerges through the mouth, it is preferable to bring it out through the nose. A well-lubricated nasopharyngeal tube is advanced through the nostril. The endoscopist grasps the tip of this tube in the posterior oropharynx with forceps or the index finger and pulls it out through the mouth. The tip of the NBC is threaded through the oral end of the

nasopharyngeal tube until it exits through the nasal end. While the GI assistant holds tightly to the NBC emerging from the esophagus, the nasopharyngeal tube is slowly pulled out through the nostril, thus bringing the tip of the NBC out through the nostril (Fig. 8.7). The nasopharyngeal tube is then discarded. The NBC is taped to the cheek or forehead of the patient, and its tip is connected to a drainage bag (Fig. 8.8).

FOLLOW-UP/COMPLICATIONS

Within 2 to 4 hrs of the procedure, the patient may be allowed to take a soft diet. The NBC is well tolerated after 1 or 2 days. NBC placement poses no additional complications other than those with ERCP and ES. Some of the minor problems associated with the NBC include nasal irritation, sore throat, or abdominal discomfort which can be managed by proper care of the nostril using throat lozenges and mild analgesics.

Plugging of the lumen and displacement into the duodenum are two rarely seen problems. Bile drainage through the NBC is an indication of the patency and proper positioning of the NBC. Occasionally mucus may plug the side holes of the NBC. This can be prevented by irrigating the NBC with 10 mL of sterile saline every 3 to 4 hrs. To ensure patency following irrigation, an attempt should be made to withdraw bile using the same syringe. Sometimes blockage of the NBC may be the result of a kink in the catheter and irrigation or withdrawal of bile may be difficult. To straighten the kink, a guidewire may be passed through the entire NBC under fluoroscopic control, followed by irrigation. If this fails, the NBC has to be replaced with a new one.

BILIARY ENDOPROSTHESIS

Endoscopic placement of stents or endoprostheses for decompression of extrahepatic biliary tree obstruction is a low-risk alternative to operative or percutaneous transhepatic decompression in patients with unresectable tumor of the pancreas or bile ducts. In addition, endoscopic biliary drainage has fewer major complications, a decreased incidence of procedure-related mortality, and a reduced number of hospital days when compared to the traditional methods of relieving bile duct obstruction.

The earlier models of endoprostheses were 5F or 7F in diameter, with a pigtail curl on each end. These stents could be introduced through a lateral-viewing

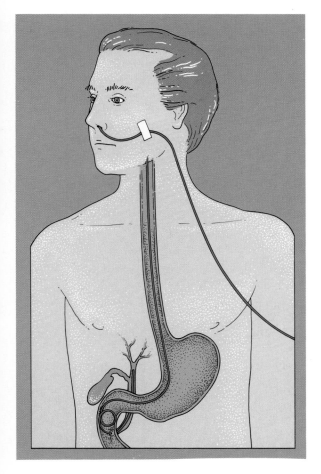

FIGURE 8.8 The proper placement of an NBC in the biliary tree. Note the tip of the NBC is in the common hepatic duct. A small loop in the duodenum helps to prevent displacement of the catheter. The remaining portion of the NBC courses through the duodenum, stomach and esophagus and is rather straight. The catheter, exiting through the nostril, is anchored to the patient's cheek with tape.

endoscope with an external diameter of 11 mm and an instrument channel size of 2.8 mm. The small caliber stent provided inadequate drainage in many cases. The rate of flow through a tube is directly proportional to its length and to the fourth power of its radius. Therefore, a small increase in the internal diameter of the stent results in a large increase in the flow rate. The configuration of the endoprosthesis is also a determining factor of the flow rate. For example, the flow rate through a straight endoprosthesis is more rapid than through a pigtail prosthesis of a similar size. Application of these concepts led to the evolution of newer model stents that achieve adequate biliary decompression. Larger lateral-viewing endoscopes with channels of 3.7 and 4.2 mm are now available, and it is possible to introduce a biliary stent of 12F diameter in addition to a 7F, 10F, and 11.5F using a 4.2 mm channel scope.

Proper positioning and anchoring are also essential for good prosthesis function. Although the pigtail curl facilitates anchoring, barbs located on either end of a straight endoprosthesis serve this purpose as well as allowing better drainage. The newest modification of these straight stents is a slight curve to conform to the anatomy of the bile duct. Wall stents, the latest addition, is made of mettalic wire mesh. This self-expandable stent anchors very well on the bile duct wall.

INDICATIONS

The major indication for biliary endoprosthesis is obstructive jaundice in patients with malignant strictures who are at high risk for an operative procedure. In this group of patients, endoprosthesis provides a cost-effective alternative to operative drainage, with relatively little morbidity and mortality from the procedure. Endoprostheses may also be used in patients with postoperative strictures, sclerosing cholangitis, retained common bile duct stones, periampullary neoplasms, bile leak, and bil-

---

TABLE 8.2 INDICATIONS FOR BILIARY ENDOPROSTHESIS

Malignant Stricture of the Bile Duct
- Primary
- Metastatic

Benign stricture of the bile duct

Periampullary neoplasm
- Inoperable
- Metastatic
- For preoperative decompression

Sclerosing cholangitis

Common bile duct stone in high operative risk patients—following unsuccessful stone extraction

Biliary fistula

Bile leak

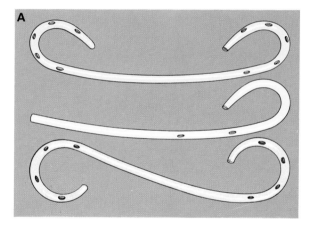
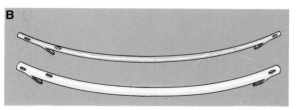

FIGURE 8.9 Endoprostheses are available in different sizes and shapes. They may have a single pigtail curl at one end or a double pigtail, one on each end (**A**). The straight Amsterdam stents (**B**) are provided with a barb on either end to anchor them in the bile duct.

iary fistula (Table 8.2). Endoprostheses may prevent recurrence in patients with postoperative biliary stricture following balloon dilatation. In this situation the endoprosthesis may be left in place for 4 to 6 months. In certain cases of sclerosing cholangitis with stricture of the extrahepatic bile ducts, an endoprosthesis may maintain biliary decompression following ES and balloon dilatation of narrowed segments. On rare occasions, in an elderly high operative risk patient in whom ES has been unsuccessful, an endoprosthesis may be the only method to avoid stone impaction in the ampulla with recurrent episodes of cholangitis. Although most patients with periampullary neoplasm are best manged by tumor resection, in patients with obvious metastases or in those at high operative risk, an endoprosthesis traversing the obstruction can provide palliative therapy. Preoperative endoprosthesis drainage in obstructive jaundice might decrease complications associated with high bilirubin levels. Bile leak resulting from bile duct injury, especially in patients who underwent laproscopic cholecystectomy, can also be managed by an endoprosthesis. The stent in this situation will prevent bile leak as well as stricture formation.

EQUIPMENT

In addition to the standard lateral-viewing endoscope with an internal instrument channel size of 2.8 mm, large-channel lateral-viewing endoscopes of 3.7 and 4.2 mm should be available for this procedure.

Endoprostheses are available in three different styles:
- The single pigtail type with a pigtail curl only at one end.
- The double pigtail stent with two pigtail curls, one at each end.
- The barbed or Amsterdam stents with a flap or barb, instead of a curl, near each end that anchors the endoprosthesis in place. In addition to the hole on either tip, the Amsterdam stents have a single side hole at the proximal tip and two side holes at the distal tip (Fig. 8.9).

The diameter of an endoprosthesis may vary from 5F to 12F, and the length as measured between the barbs may be 5 to 15 cm. Some endoprosthesis are provided with multiple side holes to faciliatate biliary drainage. Longer S-shaped stents which may occasionally be useful in bifurcation strictures. Because of the multiple bends in these stents, they can conform to the anatomy of the biliary tract (Fig. 8.10). A self-

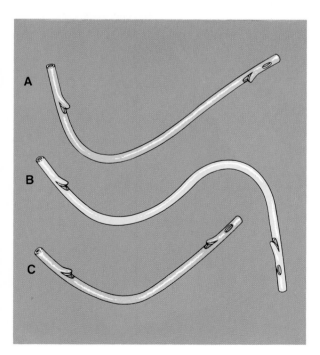

FIGURE 8.10 The newer model endoprostheses can be inserted into the left (A) or right (B) hepatic duct or into a tortuous common bile duct (C). Note that the body of these endoprostheses are curved to conform to the anatomical curves or unusual bends in the duct.

The elevator on the endoscope is closed to enable the endoscopist to feel the impact of the endoprosthesis at the elevator. When this occurs, the elevator is opened and the endoprosthesis can be visualized exiting from the endoscope (Fig. 8.17). This is a crucial time and the endoscopist should make every effort to keep the duodenoscope steady, with its tip close to the papilla. Fluoroscopic monitoring is carried out to make sure the guidewire is straight. Close endoscopic monitoring is continued so that the guidewire and guide catheter do not form a loop in the duodenum. If a small loop is formed, the guidewire and guide catheter must be withdrawn by the endoscopist to undo the loop formation. The endoprosthesis is advanced into the common bile duct and through the stricture (Fig. 8.18) by a combination of pushing on the pusher tube and upward movement with the elevator as the GI assistant maintains tension on the catheter.

The ideal position of the endoprosthesis is for the proximal barb to be located at least 1 to 2 cm above the superior margin of the stricture. The distal end of the endoprosthesis should protrude 1 cm into the duodenum, with the barb preferably at the level of the pa-

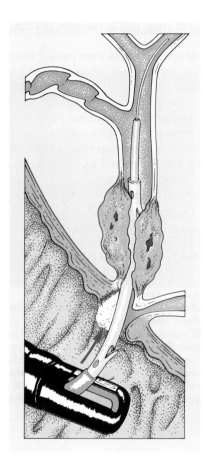

FIGURE 8.17
To advance a prosthesis through a stricture, the guidewire is introduced into the left hepatic duct. The guide catheter is positioned well above the upper margin of the stricture. The prosthesis is slowly pushed into the stricture by the pusher tube (green) that emerges from the biopsy channel of the lateral-viewing scope. The proximal barb should be about 1 cm above the superior margin of the stricture and the distal barb protrudes 1 cm into the duodenum.

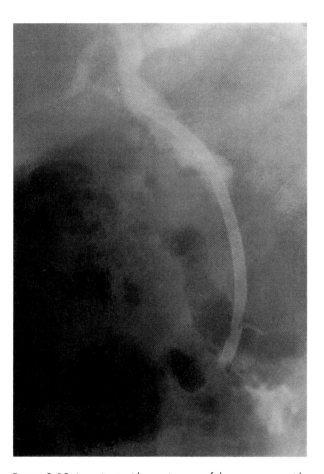

FIGURE 8.18 A patient with carcinoma of the pancreas with obstruction of the common bile duct. An Amsterdam stent has been placed across the malignant stricture. The proximal tip of the stent is in the hepatic duct while the distal end is protruding into the duodenum.

pilla. When a double pigtail stent is used, one pigtail curl should ideally be located above the obstruction and the other curl in the duodenum near the papilla (Fig. 8.19). Once these criteria are satisfied, the guide catheter and guidewire are removed. This maneuver will separate the endoprosthesis from the pusher tube (Fig. 8.20). Bile mixed with contrast medium may be seen immediately escaping through the endoprosthesis (Fig. 8.21). If the endoprosthesis slips down into the duodenum, it may be pushed back into the bile duct with the pusher tube or the tip of the endoscope.

This coaxial introducing technique using the guidewire and the guide catheter to form the axis along which the endoprosthesis is pushed into position seems to be the easiest way of placing an endoprosthesis. Figure 8.22 shows final proper siting of an endoprosthesis through a stricture.

PROSTHESIS FOLLOW-UP/COMPLICATIONS
Following the placement of the endoprosthesis, the patient may be observed in the hospital for 48 to 72 hrs. Most patients will tolerate a soft diet within 6 hrs

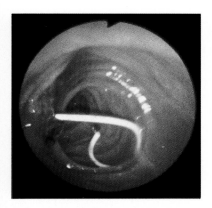

FIGURE 8.19
Endoscopic picture showing the pigtail curl of a stent protruding into the duodenum.

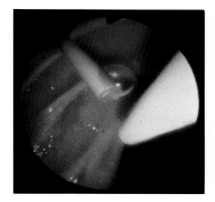

FIGURE 8.20
Endoscopic image showing the stent being separated from the pusher tube as soon as the guide catheter and the guidewire are pulled out.

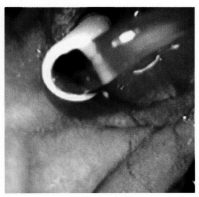

FIGURE 8.21
Endoscopic picture showing bile mixed with contrast draining through the endoprosthesis.

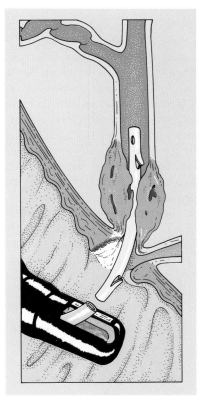

FIGURE 8.22
An endoprosthesis has been inserted through a malignant stricture of the bile duct, bridging the stricture. The guidewire and the guide catheter have been removed and the pusher tube is seen retracting into the endoscope.

of the procedure. In the presence of fever and infection, intravenous antibiotics may be continued for 24 to 48 hrs.

Experience in several centers has shown that an endoprosthesis can be placed in about 80% of patients. Failure to properly place an endoprosthesis is most commonly due either to tumors involving the papilla of Vater, in which case the bile duct orifice cannot be identified, or to neoplasms involving the hilum of the liver, causing a tight stricture of the intrahepatic ducts.

An adequately placed endoprosthesis leads to rapid correction of jaundice and the patient may be discharged from the hospital after 48 hrs of observation, to be followed on an outpatient basis. Recurrence of jaundice is usually associated with clogging of the endoprosthesis and requires stent replacement.

Complications associated with the endoprosthesis can be classified into those associated with ES (refer to Chapter 7) and those particular to the endoprosthesis, which may be immediate or delayed. Immediate complications, which are extremely rare, include bleeding, infection, or trauma to the biliary tract or duodenum. Infection or cholangitis are virtually always due to improper placement of endoprosthesis and can be treated by intravenous antibiotics while attempting to replace the stent endoscopically or by percutaneous methods.

Recurrent jaundice constitutes the most common delayed complication and is usually due to clogging of the endoprosthesis. Migration of the stent either into the common bile duct or into the duodenum can lead to recurrent cholangitis, duodenal ulcer, or perforation. Rarely jaundice may be due to tumor growth along the prosthesis or metastatic spread of a malignant tumor to the liver. Another delayed complication is erosion of the duodenal wall by the stent with ulcer formation or duodenal perforation. This particular complication is almost always due to a segment of stent protruding too far into the duodenum and rubbing against the wall.

An endoprosthesis that remains in the bile duct for more than 6 months will occasionally break. The distal portion of the stent usually will be passed through the intestine unnoticed by the patient—the remaining portion may remain in the biliary tree above the obstruction. This retained portion of the stent may be difficult to remove. This complication may be avoided by replacing the endoprosthesis at 4 to 6 month intervals.

Duodenal obstruction secondary to extrinsic compression by a growing pancreatic or periampullary carcinoma can also plug the prosthesis.

UNUSUAL PROBLEMS

The location and the diameter of the stricture are the two key factors to consider in placing an endoprosthesis. Generally, strictures closer to the ampulla of Vater allow easier placement of endoprosthesis than strictures near the porta hepatis. High-grade strictures may not permit a large endoprosthesis but may be dilated with specially devised guide catheters which are more rigid and have tapered tips. After dilatation, an appropriate endoprosthesis may be placed through the stricture segment. Dilatation using a Gruntzig balloon is rarely necessary prior to placement of an endoprosthesis. An unusually tortuous bile duct may occasionally pose difficulty for endoprosthesis placement, but the newer models of prostheses might overcome this difficulty. Some tight strictures may not permit a large endoprosthesis to be introduced, in which case the only option consists of placing a small-caliber prosthesis. Two or more small-caliber endoprostheses may sometimes be placed side-by-side (Fig. 8.23).

TIPS ON GUIDEWIRE MANIPULATIONS

Advancing the guidewire through the stricture constitutes the key step for successful stent placement. Since malignancy often leads to irregular strictures with unpredictable configurations, traversing the stricture can at times be difficult if not impossible. Some of the manipulations helpful in these situations are:

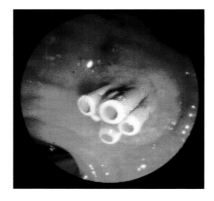

FIGURE 8.23 Occasionally, two or more endoprostheses may be placed side-by-side, as seen in this patient.

- Changing patient position.
- Using different types of guidewires.
- Coordinating guidewire manipulation along with catheter manipulations.

PATIENT POSITION

The position of the bile duct harboring the stricture is rather constant. Thus, little can be done to alter its orientation. The usual position for ERCP and related therapeutic procedures is the classical flat on the abdomen/prone position. In this position, the guidewire and catheters have a natural tendency to head toward the right hepatic duct. This is largely due to the following anatomical peculiarities:

- The long axis of the right hepatic duct is more closely aligned to the long axis of the common hepatic duct.
- The right hepatic duct lies more posteriorly, which is in alignment of the posterior location of the common bile duct.
- The right hepatic duct courses through the liver for a distance of 3 to 4 cm before it bifurcates. Advancing the guidewire into the left hepatic duct is usually difficult.

If a dominant stricture is located in the left hepatic duct, the guidewire should be advanced into the left hepatic duct. Shifting patient position laterally and anteriorly might help to negotiate the left hepatic duct.

GUIDEWIRES

The standard 0.035 in. guidewire with a long flexible tip should be used initially. If, after multiple attempts this guidewire fails to traverse the stricture, either a glidewire or torquable guidewire may be used. If advancement of the guidewire is still unsuccessful, a movable core guidewire, J- or Z-guidewire may be tried, although these guidewires are more useful in bifurcation strictures. If all these attempts fail, one may proceed with a combined procedure.

MANIPULATION OF GUIDEWIRES AND GUIDE CATHETERS

It is preferable to start cannulation of the bile duct with a guide catheter containing a standard flexible tip guidewire for stent placement. Initially an attempt is made to traverse the stricture with the catheter con-

taining the guidewire. The catheter, if at all possible, should be advanced through the stricture. If this step fails, the guide catheter may be stationed below the stricture and the guidewire advanced into it. Once the guidewire traverses the stricture segment, the guide catheter is slid over the guidewire.

This manipulation may not be successful. One of the most common reasons for failure to introduce the guidewire into the stricture zone seems to be the irregularity of the stricture. The guidewire tip may be deflected downward by a shelf-like tumor mass and thus away from the orifice of the stricture lumen. In this situation, the guide catheter should be stationed close to the orifice of the stricture lumen or at its lower end. Next, the guidewire is advanced by a few mm increments followed by the guide catheter. These manipulations, simulating the locomotion of a centipede, is continued until the entire stricture segment is traversed.

Another reason for unsuccessful introduction of the guidewire is asymmetric location of the stricture itself. The stricture may be located more toward the side of the bile duct and not necessarily in the center. Evaluation of the cholangiogram is extremely helpful under these circumstances. The guidewire may be slowly advanced into the bile duct until it is impacted against the bile duct containing the tumor mass away from the opening of the stricture (Fig. 8.24). With continued forward pressure, the guidewire will bend upon itself, forming a loop with its tip heading toward the opposite side where the narrowed lumen of the stricture is located. Keeping the guide catheter away from the tip of the guidewire but inside the bile duct, the loop formation is allowed until the guidewire is in alignment with the orifice of the stricture. Next, the guidewire is slowly withdrawn with simultaneous advancement of the guide catheter. Quite often the guidewire may engage itself into the lower portion of the stricture zone. Keeping pressure at the guide catheter, the guidewire may be further advanced through the stricture zone followed by the guide catheter. The forward movement of the guide catheter should be cautiously and carefully coordinated with withdrawal of the guidewire under constant fluoroscopic monitoring and of the memorization of stricture anatomy. Communication between the endoscopist, GI assistant, and radiographer is essential.

Occasionally a malignant stricture may be dilated using a balloon before a large prosthesis can be successfully placed.

EQUIPMENT

Gruntzig dilating balloons are constructed of a specially treated polyethylene to increase their strength and minimize stretching. Balloons range from 2 to 20 mm in diameter and 2 to 8 cm in length (Fig. 8.34). Generally, balloons 4 to 10 mm in diameter are most useful in the pancreaticobiliary tract. The balloon is attached to a 180 to 200 cm long double lumen catheter with a 1.5 cm tapered tip.

The guidewire used in conjunction with the NBC or endoprosthesis can be used to correctly place balloon catheters.

TECHNIQUE

An adequate cholangiogram is obtained using a regular cannula and is carefully reviewed for the size and location of the stricture (Fig. 8.35). Based on the anatomy of the stricture, an appropriate balloon is selected. The regular cannula is cleared of the contrast medium by injecting 5 to 10 mL of saline. A guidewire, well lubricated with silicone, is threaded into the cannula and advanced well beyond the stricture zone (Fig. 8.36). With the guidewire in position, the cannula is

withdrawn. Fluoroscopic monitoring is continued while the cannula is withdrawn to ensure that the guidewire does not slip down.

The selected balloon should be longer than the stricture. The balloon's external surface is well-lubricated and carefully threaded into the instrument channel of the lateral-viewing endoscope to avoid tearing. Compressing the balloon with the index finger and thumb facilitates passage of the folded balloon into the instrument channel. The endoscopist slowly advances the balloon while the GI assistant keeps tension on the guidewire. Care should be taken to prevent the balloon from becoming stuck in the elevator as it escapes from the endoscope by gently moving the elevator up to direct the balloon into the bile duct. The balloon is then stationed across the stricture (Fig. 8.37). Its position is confirmed by fluoroscopically observing the radiopaque markers on the balloon (Fig. 8.38). When the stricture is located near the papilla, a portion of the inflated balloon may be visible endoscopically (Fig. 8.39). An inflation pressure of 4 to 6 atm is applied for 30 sec on three successive occasions using a 20 mL syringe filled with 30% Renografin. When fully inflated, the balloon assumes a dumbbell shape because of the circumferential pressure exerted at the stricture zone. Following dilatation, the balloon is bled of contrast medium and with-

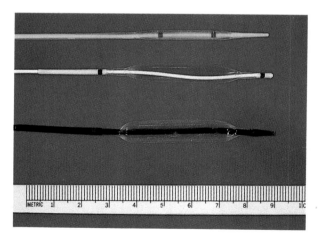

FIGURE 8.34 The diameter of an inflated Gruntzig balloon can be (from the top) 4, 8 or 10 mm. The catheter containing the balloon can be 8F or 5F. A 4 mm balloon is useful to dilate a very tight stricture.

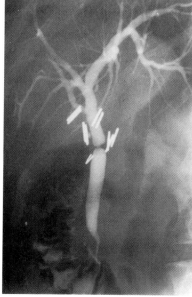

FIGURE 8.35 Cholangiogram showing a stricture involving the common hepatic duct with minimal dilatation of the intrahepatic duct.

ENDOSCOPIC MANAGEMENT OF BILIARY TRACT OBSTRUCTION

drawn through the endoscope. The balloon is twisted counterclockwise as it is withdrawn from the endoscope to preserve its fold orientation for future insertions.

BALLOON DILATATION—FOLLOW-UP/ COMPLICATIONS

Balloon dilatation in most instances enhances biliary drainage. Objectively, successful balloon dilatation is associated with a widened diameter of the strictured zone and a more rapid contrast drainage from the common bile duct (Fig. 8.40). Clinical improvement in jaundice and a drop in serum bilirubin may be observed in 24 to 48 hrs following balloon dilatation. A decrease in the incidence of cholangitis is observed in most patients.

Complications occur in approximately 10% of patients, of which the most serious are pancreatitis and injury to the bile duct. Almost every case of pancreatitis following balloon dilatation responds to conservative management. Laceration of the bile duct may be immediately identified by contrast medium extravasating beyond the confines of the biliary tree. In most instances this complication will resolve spontaneously if the lacerated area is bridged by an endoprosthesis.

The success rate of balloon dilatation depends on the number, severity, and location of strictures. Multiple strictures, strictures near the hilum of the liver, and very tight strictures may respond poorly to this therapeutic modality. The long-term results of balloon dilatation of benign strictures are unknown.

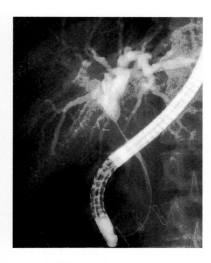

FIGURE 8.36 A guidewire is seen advancing through the stricture segment in the intrahepatic duct.

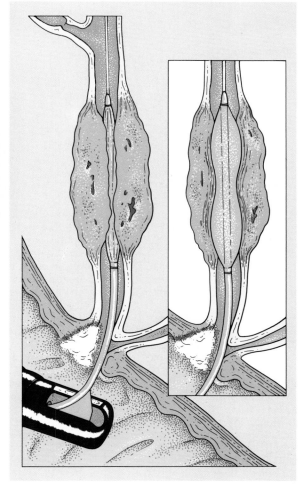

FIGURE 8.37 A guidewire is passed through the stricture up to the hepatic duct. The balloon catheter is advanced over the guidewire and stationed through the strictured segment. The Gruntzig balloon is slowly inflated (inset) exerting a radial force on the stricture and resulting in its dilatation. When the balloon is fully inflated and under pressure from the stricture mass, it assumes a dumbbell shape.

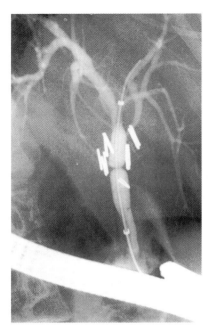

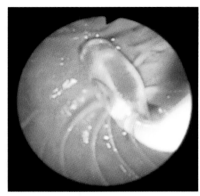

FIGURE 8.39 Endoscopic view during biliary duct dilatation in a patient who had stricture involving the distal common bile duct. A portion of the inflated balloon is visible through the papillary orifice.

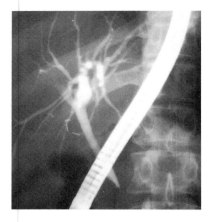

FIGURE 8.40 Cholangiogram following balloon dilatation of the patient shown in Figure 8.36. Note that the stricture segment (between the clips) is dilated and has an almost normal diameter.

FIGURE 8.38 Cholangiogram demonstrating the fully inflated Gruntzig balloon placed in the stricture segment of the same patient shown in Figure 8.35.

REFERENCES

Burcharth F, Efsen F, Christiansen LA, et al: Nonsurgical internal biliary drainage by endoprosthesis. *Surg Gynecol Obstet* 1981;153:857.

Burcharth F, Jensen LI, Oleson K: Endoprosthesis for internal drainage of the biliary tract. *Gastroenterology* 1979;77:133.

Cotton PB: Duodenoscopic placement of biliary prostheses to relieve malignant obstructive jaundice. *Br J Surg* 1982;69:501.

Foutch PG, Sivak MV Jr: Therapeutic endoscopic balloon dilatation of extrahepatic biliary ducts. *Am J Gastroenterol* 1985;80;7:575.

Geenen JE, Derfus D, Welch JM: Biliary balloon dilatation. *Endoscopy Rev* 1985;2;1:10.

Geenen DJ, Geenen JE, Hogan WJ, et al: Endoscopic therapy for benign bile duct strictures. *Gastrointest Endosc* 1989;35:367.

Hatfield ARW, Tobias R, Terblanche J et al: Preoperative external biliary drainage in obstructive jaundice. *Lancet* 1982; 2:896.

Johnson GK, Geenen JE, Venu RP, Hogan WJ: Sclerosing cholangitis: Treatment with endoscopic sphincterotomy and balloon dilatation. *Gastrointest Endosc* 1985;31:153. Abstract.

Johnson GK, Geenen JE, Venu RP, et al: Endoscopic treatment of biliary tract strictures in sclerosing cholangitis: A larger series and recommendations for treatment. *Gastrointest Endosc* 1991;37:38.

Kozarek RA: Endoscopic Gruntzig balloon dilatation of gastrointestinal stenoses. *J Clin Gastroenterol* 1984;6:401.

Siegel JH, Yatto RP: Biliary endoprostheses for management of retained common bile duct stones. *Am J Gastroenterol* 1984;79:50.

Venu RP, Geenen JE, Toouli J, et al: Gallstone dissolution using mono-octanoin infusion through an endoscopically placed nasobiliary catheter. *Am J Gastroenterol* 1982;77:227.

Venu RP, Rolny P, Geenen JE, et al: Is there a need for multiple stents in hilar strictures? *Gastrointest Endosc* 1990;36:197.

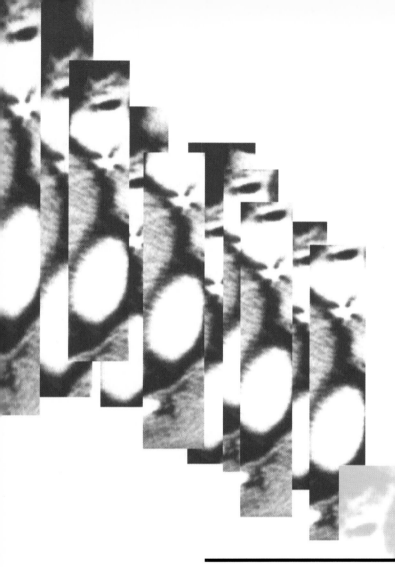

Pancreatic Endoscopy

Joseph E. Geenen, MD

9

prosthesis to protrude 1 cm into the duodenum with the barb preferably at the level of the papilla (Fig. 9.8). Once these criteria are satisfied, the guidewire is removed. This maneuver will separate the endoprosthesis from the pusher tube. If the endoprosthesis slips too far into the duodenum, it may be pushed back into the pancreatic duct with the pusher tube or the tip of the endoscope.

PROSTHESIS FOLLOWUP/COMPLICATIONS

Following placement of the endoprosthesis, the patient may be observed in the hospital for 24 to 48 hrs. Most patients will tolerate a soft diet after 12 to 24 hrs. Immediate complications following pancreatic duct stent placement include abdominal pain and mild pancreatitis. Pseudocyst formation or sepsis rarely occur following stent placement.

Long-term complications include clogging of stents in 3 to 4 months, requiring replacement. Migration of the stent into the pancreatic duct or out of the pancre-

atic duct into the duodenum occurs in approximately 5% to 10% of patients.

ENDOSCOPIC NASOPANCREATIC CATHETER PLACEMENT

Placement of an endoscopic nasopancreatic catheter (NPC) is similar to placement of a nasobiliary catheter. A nasopancreatic catheter differs from the nasobiliary catheter as it has no pigtail and has multiple side holes to drain the pancreatic side branches (Fig. 9.9).

INDICATIONS

The following are current indications for the use of nasopancreatic catheters:

* Following traumatic or repeated cannulation of the pancreatic duct.
* Post endoscopic sphincterotomy, catheter or bal-

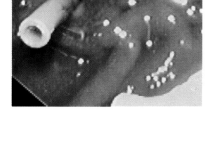

FIGURE 9.8 Endoscopic image showing tip of barbed endoprosthesis protruding into the duodenum.

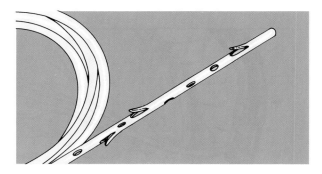

FIGURE 9.9 NPC with multiple side holes to drain pancreatic duct side branches.

loon dilation of the pancreatic duct sphincter.
• Treatment of pancreatic duct stone during extracorporeal shock-wave lithotripsy (ESWL).

EQUIPMENT

Equipment needed for nasopancreatic catheter placement includes an NPC with connecting bag and washer, guidewires of different sizes, a short nasopharyngeal or nasogastric tube, and grasping forceps.

NPCs are available in sizes 5F, 7F and 9F. These catheters can be advanced through the 3.2 or 4.2 mm instrument channel of a lateral-viewing endoscope. The NPC has a straight end with barbs to maintain its position in the pancreatic duct (Fig. 9.10 and refer to Fig. 9.9).

The standard guidewire is 480 cm long with a diameter of 0.035 in. The tip of the guidewire that negotiates the pancreatic duct is blunt and flexible. Small caliber guidewires are also available with diameters of 0.018 to 0.025 in.

Specially designed nasopharyngeal tubes are available for transpositioning NPCs through the nostrils.

They are 25 cm long and 16F in diameter. The tip that is inserted through the nostril is rounded and smooth but, unlike a standard nasogastric tube, there are no side holes. If a special nasopharyngeal tube is not available, a 16F Levine tube or nasogastric tube of any kind may be shortened to 25 to 30 cm and used for this purpose.

TECHNIQUE

Before positioning the NPC in the pancreatic duct, the endoscopist should review the pancreatogram to be familiar with the anatomy of the pancreatic duct, assessing the length and location of strictures or the size and number of stones.

The regular or ball-tipped cannula used for cannulating the pancreatic duct is carefully advanced well into the pancreatic duct (Table 9.2). The cannula should be beyond the stricture or stones. Two mL of contrast medium is instilled through the cannula to locate its tip. The cannula is then cleared of contrast by injection of 2 to 3 cc of normal saline, ensuring that contrast material will not adhere to the inner surface

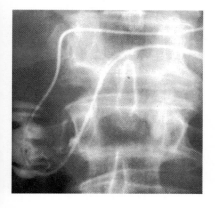

FIGURE 9.10 This patient's radiograph shows the NPC in place.

TABLE 9.2 NASOPANCREATIC CATHETER PLACEMENT (NPC) TECHNIQUE

• Cannulation of pancreatic duct with a 5F regular cannula or ball-tipped catheter
• Advancement of the guidewire through the cannula beyond the obstruction
• Withdrawal of the cannula over the guidewire
• Advancement of the NPC over the guidewire into the pancreatic duct after the guidewire is cleaned and sprayed with silicone
• Withdrawal of the endoscope over the NPC
• Transposition of the NPC through the nose
• Taping the NPC to the cheek and connecting to a drainage bag

of the cannula and cause difficulty in advancement of the guidewire.

An appropriate guidewire of 480 cm is selected for exchange. The flexible or floppy end of the guidewire is placed through the cannula and slowly advanced into the pancreatic duct. The guidewire should be kept straight by the GI assistant who, standing at a distance, holds the end of the guidewire taut. The endoscope position should be close to the papilla, preferably inferior to and looking upward toward it. Keeping the papilla in view, the endoscopist makes tip adjustments as needed to maintain the desired

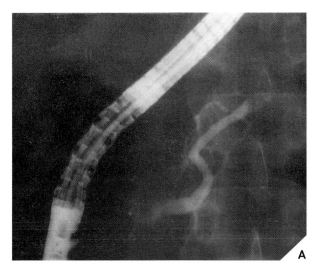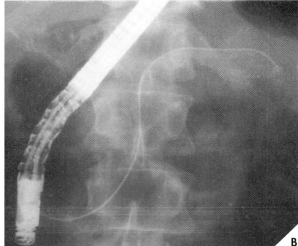

FIGURE 9.11 Radiograph showing stone in the pancreatic duct (A). Guidewire and NPC in pancreatic duct beyond a stone (B).

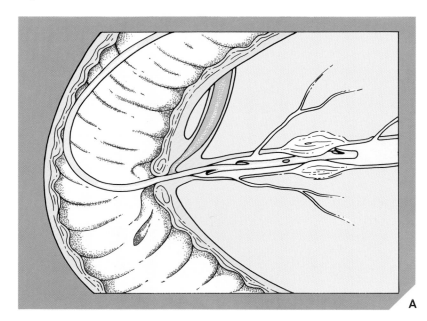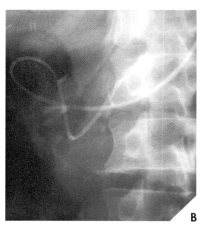

FIGURE 9.12 The NPC is placed beyond the stricture in main pancreatic duct (A). Radiograph of an NPC after placement in pancreatic duct (B). The remainder of the NPC is coursing through the duodenal bulb, pylorus, and stomach.

PANCREATIC ENDOSCOPY

angle while simultaneously observing the guidewire advancement fluoroscopically. Communication between the endoscopist and GI assistant is extremely important in coordinating each step of the procedure.

Once the guidewire has been properly sited within the pancreatic duct, close to the tail of the pancreas, the cannula is slowly removed over it. Fluoroscopy is used intermittently to verify the guidewire position.

The external portion of the guidewire is cleaned with saline and sprayed with silicone. An appropriate NPC is selected. The tapered end of the NPC is threaded over the guidewire and slowly advanced through the instrument channel of the endoscope. As the NPC exits from the endoscope, the elevator is opened so that the catheter tip will not impact on the elevator mechanism. By gentle pushing, the NPC advances steadily over the guidewire through the ampulla into the pancreatic duct. Care is taken to avoid loop formation by keeping the endoscope close to the papilla (Fig. 9.11). Once the NPC reaches the desired position in the pancreatic duct, close to the tail or beyond the stricture or stone, the guidewire is removed. The endoscope is thus slowly withdrawn over the NPC. This is accomplished by a coordinated team effort by the endoscopist, radiology technician, and GI assistant. By intermittent flu-

oroscopic observation, the radiology technician confirms that the tip of the NPC is not displaced. While the endoscopist is advancing the NPC, the GI assistant withdraws the endoscope in increments of 1 or 2 cm. This maintains the stationary position of the NPC. After the endoscope and mouthguard are removed from the patient, the entire catheter position is viewed fluoroscopically. Loops or extra length of the NPC in the throat, esophagus, stomach, or duodenum are undesirable and are straightened or removed by gently pulling on the NPC. Ideally, the tip of the NPC should be well beyond the obstruction or stone in the distal body or tail of the pancreas (Fig. 9.12).

Although the NPC normally emerges through the mouth, it is preferable to bring it out through the nose (Fig. 9.13). A well-lubricated nasopharyngeal tube is advanced through the nostril to the posterior oropharynx, where the endoscopist grasps the tip with forceps or the fingers and pulls it out through the mouth. The tip of the NPC is threaded through the oral end of the nasopharyngeal tube until it exits through the nasal end. While the GI assistant holds tightly to the NPC emerging from the esophagus, the nasopharyngeal tube with the attached NPC tip is slowly pulled out through the nostril. The nasopharyngeal tube is then discarded. The NPC is taped to the cheek or forehead

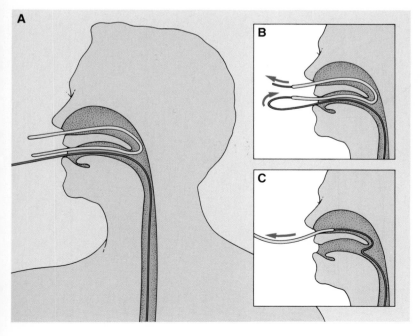

FIGURE 9.13 NPC brought out through the nose. The NPC exits through the mouth (**A**). A nasopharyngeal tube is advanced through the nose and brought out through the mouth. The NPC is then threaded through the oral end of the nasopharyngeal catheter until it passes out through the nasal end of the nasopharyngeal tube (**B**). Slow pulling on the nasopharyngeal tube will bring the NPC out through the nose (**C**).

of the patient, and the tip is connected to a drainage bag (Fig. 9.14).

Some of the minor problems associated with NPC include nasal irritation, sore throat, or abdominal discomfort, which can be managed by proper care of the nostril and using throat lozenges and mild analgesics.

ENDOSCOPIC TECHNIQUE OF DRAINAGE OF PANCREATIC PSEUDOCYSTS

A pseudocyst is not an uncommon complication of acute pancreatitis. Resolution of pancreatic pseudocysts after six weeks is uncommon. Moreover, chronic cysts greater than 5 cm have a high incidence of complications such as bleeding, infection, obstruction, and perforation. Intervention has traditionally been recommended in symptomatic or rapidly enlarging acute pseudocysts. Drainage could be achieved by the traditional surgical approach, interventional radiological approach, and most recently by the endoscopic approach.

Endoscopically, pseudocysts can be drained by:

- Transpapillary approach
- Cystoduodenostomy
- Cystogastrostomy

TECHNIQUE
It is important to define the local anatomy of a pseudocyst with a CT scan of the abdomen and/or endoscopic ultrasonogram (EUS). EUS, if available, will

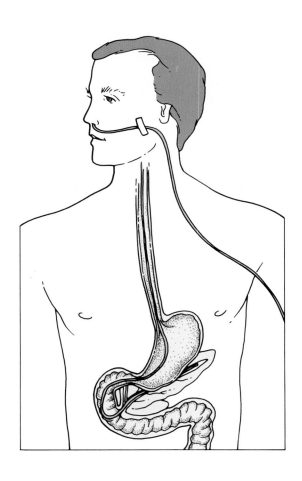

FIGURE 9.14 The proper placement of NPC in the pancreatic duct. Note the tip of NPC in the pancreatic duct. The remaining portion of NPC courses through the duodenum, stomach, and esophagus and is straight. The catheter exiting through the nostril is anchored to the patient's cheek with tape.

also help to define local vascularity and more precise pseudocyst anatomy.

CONTRAINDICATIONS TO THE ENDOSCOPIC APPROACH

Contraindications to endoscopically draining a pancreatic pseudocyst are:

- Recent intracystic bleeding and formation of pseudoaneurysm.

- Distance in excess of 1 cm between the cyst and gut wall is a relative contraindication.
- Major coagulopathy.

TRANSPAPILLARY APPROACH

This technique is most useful with small pseudocysts and ongoing disruptions in the head and body of the pancreas, particularly when such lesions do not impinge upon the stomach or duodenal wall (Fig. 9.15).

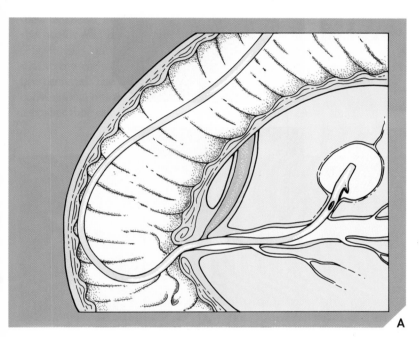

FIGURE 9.15 NPC in pseudocyst—the transpapillary approach (A). Radiograph shows NPC entering the pseudocyst through the papilla (B).

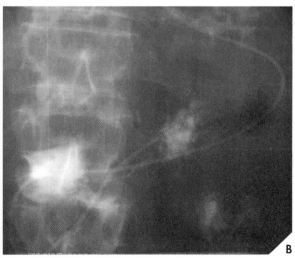

Endoscopic Sphincterotomy of Pancreatic Duct Segment

Endoscopic pancreatic sphincterotomy has generally been considered dangerous and something to avoid. However, preliminary results of pancreatic sphincterotomy have resulted in minimal problems or complications in a very select group of patients. Pancreatic sphincterotomy may be acceptably safe in chronic pancreatitis, but may be extremely hazardous in papillary stenosis. It is most commonly performed after a bile duct sphincterotomy, and in most situations, a stent is placed in the pancreatic duct to prevent its obstruction at the papillary orifice by swelling or edema.

Indications
The following are indications for endoscopic sphincterotomy of the pancreatic duct segment:

- Papillary stenosis with elevated basal SO pressure in pancreatic duct segment after biliary sphincterotomy
- To permit diagnostic or therapeutic procedures—
    Large stent for tumor or stricture
    Pancreatic stone removal
    Intraductal radiation therapy
    Pancreatoscopy

Technique
Pancreatic sphincterotomy may be performed using a short wire, standard or precut sphincterotome. Also a needle-knife papillotome may be used over a pancreatic duct stent. In most patients, a bile duct sphincterotomy had been performed at an earlier date. A 3 to 4 mm incision is made between the 12 and 1 o'clock position toward the common bile duct opening using standard electrocautery setting (Fig. 9.20). A stent or NPC should be placed across the incised sphincter for at least 24 hrs to help prevent pancreatitis.

Complications
Mild pancreatitis occurs in 8% to 10% of patients following pancreatic sphincterotomy. The incidence of pancreatitis will be higher in patients with a normal pancreas. Pseudocyst may occur in approximately 2% of patients.

Balloon Dilatation

Balloon dilatation is rarely performed in diseases of the pancreas. More often, stenosis of the papilla or strictures of the pancreatic duct are dilated with dilating graduated catheters or Soehendra catheters.

Gruntzig Balloon Dilatation for Pancreatic Duct Stricture–Indications
The technique of luminal dilatation using a Gruntzig balloon was initially performed for occlusive vascular disorders. Angioplastic balloon dilatation has become an integral part of therapeutic endoscopy for biliary tract stricture. The same technique has been applied for balloon dilatation of pancreatic duct stricture.

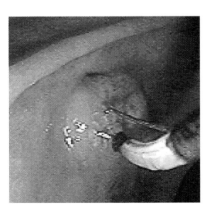

Figure 9.20 Precut sphincterome is inserted into pancreatic duct with wire oriented toward CBD opening at 12 o'clock

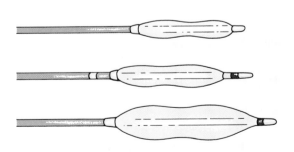

Figure 9.21 The diameter of an inflated Gruntzig balloon can be (from the top) 4 , 6, or 8 mm and 2 to 4 cm in length.

This procedure is indicated when there is:

- Papillary stenosis or stricture of pancreatic sphincter.
- Stricture in main pancreatic duct.

EQUIPMENT

Gruntzig dilatating balloons are constructed of a specially treated polyethylene material to increase their strength and minimize stretching. Balloons range from 4 to 10 mm in diameter and 2 to 4 cm in length (Fig. 9.21). Generally, balloons 4 mm in diameter are most useful in the pancreatic duct. The balloon is attached to a 180 to 200 cm long, double-lumen catheter with a 1.5 cm tapered tip.

The guidewire used in conjunction with NPC or endoprosthesis can be used to achieve correct placement of balloon catheters.

TECHNIQUE

An adequate pancreatogram through major or minor papilla, depending on the clinical situation, is performed and carefully reviewed for the size and location of stricture (Fig. 9.22A). Based on the anatomy of the stricture, an appropriate balloon is selected. The cannula is cleared of the contrast medium by injecting 2 to 3 mL of saline. A guidewire, well-lubricated with silicone, is threaded into the cannula and advanced well beyond the stricture (Fig. 9.22B). With the guidewire in position, the cannula is withdrawn. Fluoroscopic monitoring is continued while the cannula is withdrawn to ensure that the guidewire does not move.

The balloon selected should be longer than the stricture. The external surface of the balloon is well lubricated and carefully threaded into the instru-

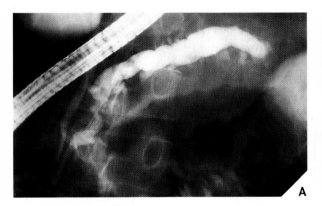

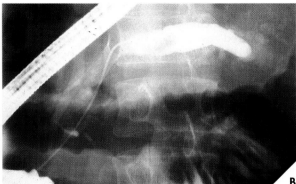

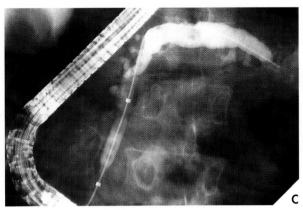

FIGURE 9.22 In this patient's pancreatogram, note the pancreatic duct stricture in the head of the pancreas (A). The guidewire is seen advancing through the stricture segment beyond the stone in the pancreatic duct (B). The Gruntzig balloon is placed in the stricture segment and fully inflated (C).

COMPLICATIONS

Complications include bleeding, acute pancreatitis, and rarely retroperitoneal perforation from endoscopic sphincterotomy. Almost all these complications can be treated medically.

REFERENCES

Cremer M, Deviere J, Delhaye M, et al: Non-surgical management of severe chronic pancreatitis. Scand J Gastroenterol 1990;25(suppl 175):74.

Cremer M, Deviere J, Engelholm: Endoscopic management of cysts and pseudocysts in chronic pancreatitis: Long term follow-up after 7 years of experience. Gastrointest Endosc 1989;35:1.

Fuji T, Amarao R, Ohmura T, et al: Endoscopic pancreatic sphincterotomy technique and evaluation. Endoscopy 1989;21:27.

Geenen JE: ASGE Distinguished Lecture—Endoscopic therapy of pancreatic disease: A new horizon. Gastrointest Endosc 1988;34;5:386.

Grimm H, Meyer WH, Nam VCH, Soehendra N: New modalities for treating chronic pancreatitis. Endoscopy 1989;21:70.

Huibregtse K, Scheider B, Vrij AA, et al: Endoscopic pancreatic drainage in chronic pancreatitis. Gastrointest Endosc 1988;34:9.

Kozarek RA, Ball TJ, Patterson DJ, et al: Endoscopic transpapillary therapy for disrupted pancreatic duct and pseudocyst. Gastrointest Endosc 1990;36:203.

Kozarek RA, Patterson DJ, Ball TS, et al: Endoscopic placement of pancreatic stents and drains in the management of pancreatitis. Ann Surg 1989;209:261.

Lehman G, O'Connor K, Toiano L, et al: Endoscopic papillotomy and stenting of the minor papilla in pancreas divisum. Gastrointest Endosc 1989;35:167.

McCarthy J, Geenen JE, Hogan WJ: Preliminary experience with endoscopic stent placement in benign pancreatic disease. Gastrointest Endosc 1988;34:16.

Prabhu M, Geenen JE, Hogan WJ, et al: Role of endoscopic stent placement in the treatment of acute recurrent pancreatitis associated with pancreas divisum. Gastrointest Endosc 1989;2:165.

Sahel J, Bastid C, Pellat B, et al: Endoscopic cystoduodenostomy of cysts of chronic calcifying pancreatitis. A report of 20 cases. Pancreas 1987;2:447.

Siegel JH, Pullano WJ, Safrany L: Endoscopic sphincterotomy for acquired pancreatitis: Effective long term management. Gastrointest Endosc 1989;35:168.

Siegel JH, Ben-Zvi JS, Pullano W, et al: Effectiveness of endoscopic drainage for pancreas divisum: Endoscopic and surgical results in 31 patients. Endoscopy 1990;22:129.

Gastrointestinal
Polypectomy

Jerome D. Waye, MD

10

INTRODUCTION

The term **polyp** refers to any abnormal protuberance on the surface of a mucous membrane. Polyps may be caused by inflammation, leiomyomas, lipomas, or they may be neoplasms.

There are two basic types of polyps (Fig. 10.1):

- Pedunculated polyps are attached to the intestinal wall by a stalk. The pedicles may vary in length and thickness (Figs. 10.2, 10.3).
- Sessile polyps, which are attached to the intestinal wall directly, arise from the mucosa in a variety of ways. Those that are less than 8 mm in diameter almost invariably have the shape of a split pea. Polyps greater than 8 mm in diameter can assume one of several configurations.

The **marble-type** polyp has a fairly narrow base, and resembles a round marble. These polyps are attached to the colon wall by a small connection, which is considerably narrower than the polyp's widest diameter (Fig. 10.4).

The **mountain-type** polyp is well-defined, often multilobulated, and the edges can be distinctly seen; the base is frequently the widest part of the polyp (Fig. 10.5).

The **clamshell** polyp is wrapped around a colon fold; a polyp of this type is often difficult to visualize completely because part of its attachment is on the opposite side of the fold (Fig. 10.6).

The **carpet** polyp is a relatively flat adenoma that may extend laterally over a wide area. The limits of the polyp are often difficult to assess, because its edges blend into the surrounding mucosa (Figs. 10.7, 10.8).

Extended polyps have a combination of attachments; the major component is usually a mountain or clamshell type. The edges of the polyp extend diffusely into the mucosa (Fig. 10.9).

Removal of polyps with a wire loop technique requires the use of two simultaneous modalities:

- Guillotine force generated by retraction of the wire into its plastic sheath.
- Thermal energy to heat seal nutrient blood vessels.
- The role of these factors will be discussed.

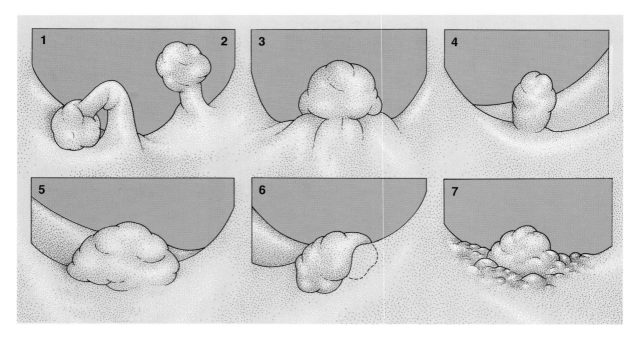

FIGURE 10.1 Schematic representation of polyp types. 1, Pedunculated polyp on a long pedicle; **2,** pedunculated polyp; **3,** polyp with pseudopedicle; **4,** marble-type polyp; **5,** mountain-type polyp; **6,** clamshell polyp; **7,** extended polyp consisting of carpet polyp with large sessile component.

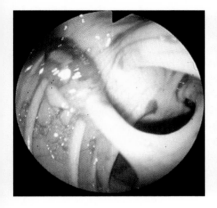

FIGURE 10.2 Typical tubular adenoma on a long, slender pedicle. This pedunculated polyp is found in the area of the hepatic flexure.

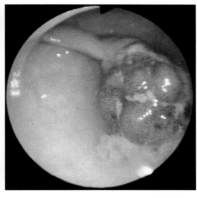

FIGURE 10.3 Multilobulated pedunculated polyp with hemorrhagic areas on its tip.

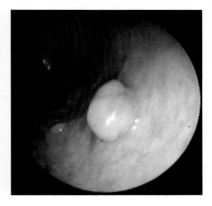

FIGURE 10.4 Two polyps. The larger one is a typical marble-type whose base is smaller than its maximum diameter. The smaller one is diminutive.

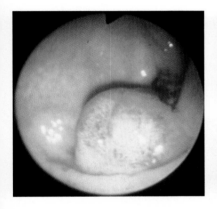

FIGURE 10.5 This mountain-type polyp has a base as broad as its maximum diameter.

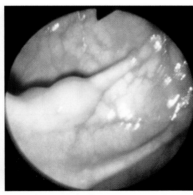

FIGURE 10.6 Clamshell configuration. This tubular adenoma is wrapped around a fold in the colon.

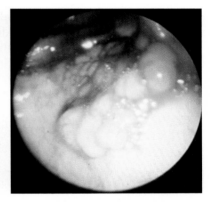

FIGURE 10.7 Broad-based, flat, carpet-type lesion, with multiple larger projections.

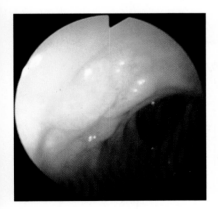

FIGURE 10.8 Carpet configuration: Note the small bumpy nodules.

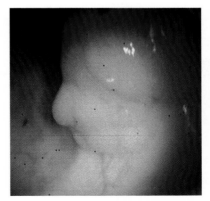

FIGURE 10.9 Multiple small frond-like components are seen on the colon wall, associated with a large mountain-type polyp. This combination is called an extended polyp.

INDICATIONS FOR RESECTION

Theoretically, all polyps are abnormal and should be removed. However, polyps less than 1 cm in diameter rarely produce bleeding, and infrequently contain malignancy.

All polyps greater than 1 cm should be resected. There is controversy about whether small colon polyps found on radiographic study should prompt a colonoscopic examination and polypectomy. The decision for endoscopy should be based on the patient's age, family history, past medical history, presence of other diseases, and the knowledge that most small colon polyps are adenomas.

MALIGNANCY

While it may not be possible to correctly identify the histologic pathology of any polyp by its gross visual appearance, there are several visual clues to malignancy (Figs. 10.10–10.13). Tubular adenomas are usually red, with a smooth surface, but there may be well-defined nodulations, like knuckles protruding from a closed fist. The villous adenoma is also red and is rarely found as a tiny polyp, since the villous component appears to be a differentiation associated with maturation of some adenomas. The surface of a villous adenoma is usually not smooth, but resembles a head of cauliflower. Tubulovillous adenomas, being a mixture, have configurations of both types.

It may be impossible to visually identify which adenomas are or will become malignant, although it is known that the incidence of malignancy increases in proportion to the degree of the villous component of the adenoma. Cancer in an adenoma may cause surface ulceration, a variegated color of the polyp, marked irregularity of the surface, or firmness to palpation by a probe. Because malignancy in adenomas is often missed in single or even multiple forceps biopsies, histologic evaluation should be based on the entire resected lesion.

FACTORS IN THE POLYPECTOMY DECISION

The experience and expertise of the endoscopist are the primary factors in the decision to remove polyps endo-

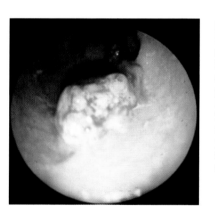

FIGURE 10.10 Polyp demonstrating one of the visual clues to carcinoma: spontaneous hemorrhages on the surface. This mountain-type polyp is a typical carcinoma of the colon.

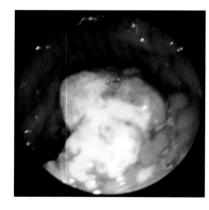

FIGURE 10.11 An irregular, waxy polyp with multiple nodulations. This is a characteristic appearance of cancer of the sigmoid colon.

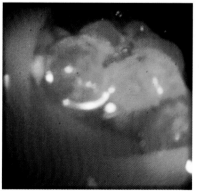

FIGURE 10.12 Malignancy in this polyp is indicated by the broad base and multilobulated appearance.

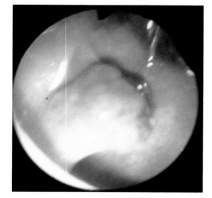

FIGURE 10.13 The irregular head with extremely short pedicle of this polyp should raise the suspicion of cancer. The entire distal end of this lesion is malignant.

scopically. The more experienced endoscopist, using excellent control of the instrument tip, may be able to shave a large polyp off the colon wall, whereas others may elect to have the polyp removed surgically.

The location of the polyp is also important. Polyps in the rectum and lower sigmoid colon can be resected more safely than those in the cecum, where the wall is thinner.

The easiest polyps to remove endoscopically are **diminutive** polyps—those less than 8 mm. These polyps can be removed with the hot-biopsy forceps, combining techniques of biopsy and electrofulguration of the polyp base, or with the wire snare and cautery method.

EQUIPMENT

Any electrosurgical unit may be used to supply thermal energy during polypectomy, and most units have solid-state circuitry, providing the operator with a choice of either cutting current, coagulation current, or a blend of both. Electrocautery current heat seals blood vessels to prevent excessive bleeding.

Most electrosurgical units do not permit precise adjustment of the amount of current applied. Therefore, it may not be possible to correlate a particular dial setting on one unit with the same setting on another unit. Electrosurgical units are not linearly calibrated, so that the energy output generated by mov-

ing the dial from 1 to 2 may not correspond to that generated by going from 3 to 4. For this reason it is important that the endoscopist become thoroughly familiar with the units available for polypectomy, and that guidelines be developed for each unit in use. Most endoscopists use pure coagulation current for polypectomy rather than blended current, and advocate using continuous application of power at a single predetermined setting.

Most polyps are removed by wire snares or with the hot biopsy forceps, which are opened and closed by a trained gastrointestinal assistant. The wire snares have insulated plastic handles, with a sliding bar mechanism for opening and closing the loop. Polypectomy snares may have considerably different cutting characteristics, depending on the composition and diameter of different wires: A thin wire will cut through tissue more quickly than a thick one.

The actual separation of a polyp from the wall is accomplished by drawing a heated wire across the area of attachment. The wire loop will not sever the polyp if it cannot be withdrawn into the tip of the plastic sheath. Because sheath shortening due to compression—to a greater or lesser extent—occurs during every polypectomy, the guillotine force required for severance can only be guaranteed by ensuring that the tip of the wire retracts inside the tip of the plastic sheath by at least 1.5 cm (Fig. 10.14). This should be tested by the assistant prior to each use of a snare. If

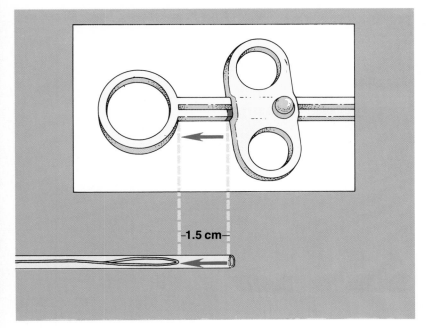

FIGURE 10.14 To prevent snare entrapment during polypectomy, the wire tip should retract into the sheath for a distance of at least 1.5 cm. Every new snare should be tested by fully closing the slide bar and measuring the distance of wire retraction.

–1.5 cm–

the 1.5 cm retractability criteria is not met, the snare has the potential for becoming stuck in the tissue during polypectomy.

The assistant should be able to mark the snare handle in such a fashion that the slide bar location indicates the point where the snare tip closes to the mouth of the sheath. This permits the endoscopy assistant to estimate the size of the captured polyp or pedicle by gauging the distance from the sliding bar to the handle mark. If that distance is greater than the endoscopist's estimate of the actual amount ensnared, normal tissue may have been trapped within the loop.

HOT-BIOPSY FORCEPS TECHNIQUE

This technique permits small sessile polyps less than 8 mm in diameter to be completely removed and recovered for biopsy with ablation of the base. The polyp is grasped between the jaws of the insulated forceps and lifted away from the intestinal wall by manipulation of the angulation controls (Fig. 10.15). This maneuver pulls the mucosa away from the submucosa and mus-

cularis propria so that application of current causes only slight heating of the deeper tissues (Fig. 10.16). With the grasped polyp pulled gently toward the lumen, coagulation current is applied. Under direct vision, a whitish area can be seen to encircle the polyp base; when this area is 1 to 2 mm wide, the current is discontinued, and the polyp pulled off its base. Some pinkish, undesiccated tissue may remain at the polypectomy site, but the base, now damaged by the current, will slough off. Withdrawal of the biopsy forceps through the instrument provides a portion of undamaged tissue for histologic evaluation.

When using the hot-biopsy forceps, it is important not to push the polyp toward the wall, since this tends to displace some of the loose areolar submucosal tissue, and may result in a deep burn to the colon wall.

WIRE SNARE AND CAUTERY TECHNIQUE

Monopolar electrocoagulation techniques are the standard and have withstood the test of time. Current

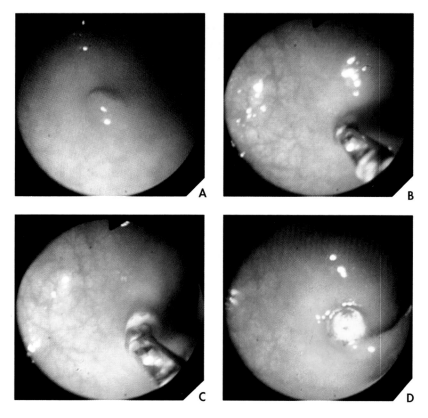

FIGURE 10.15 Technique of hot-biopsy forceps removal of a small hyperplastic polyp (A). The forceps grasp the polyp, and (B) pull it away from the colon wall. Upon application of coagulation current, a small zone of white coagulum can be seen (C). At this point current is discontinued and the forceps retracted. Frame (D) demonstrates the appearance of the polypectomy site.

GASTROINTESTINAL POLYPECTOMY

from the wire snare passes through the body tissues and is returned through a ground plate. Bipolar snares and forceps have some theoretic advantages, but they have not yet been demonstrated to be more beneficial or safer than the monopolar apparatus.

During current transfer, considerable heat is generated at the narrowest portion of tissue within the wire loop; this heat tends to cauterize blood vessels while exploding and disrupting tissue cells. Application of current in conjunction with the guillotine effect of pulling the wire loop into the plastic catheter causes the polyp to separate from its attachment. Closure of the wire loop should begin when the endoscopist sees whitening of the tissue around the loop. Observation

of tissue damage guarantees that guillotine of the polyp will not take place without adequate blood vessel cauterization.

An attempt should be made to decrease the amount of heat given to the deeper tissues of the colon during current application. This is accomplished by using the up/down control knob to raise the polyp off the wall.

Large polyps, or those with a long pedicle, may crook over, allowing a portion of the polyp head to contact the intestinal wall (Fig. 10.17). If this occurs, heat may be transferred through the alternate pathway, causing a burn of the wall adjacent to the polyp. This is a rare occurrence, which the operator should attempt to avoid. Jiggling the polyp head to and fro

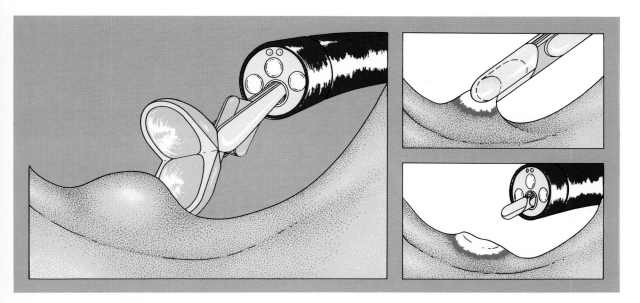

FIGURE 10.16 Hot-biopsy forceps pulling the polyp away from the submucosa, preventing thermal injury to deeper tissues.

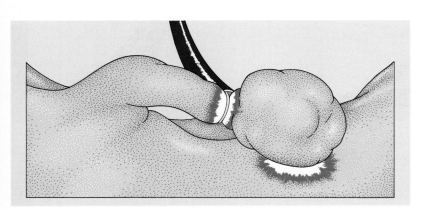

FIGURE 10.17 Pedunculated polyps may bend over so that the polyp head is in contact with the mucosa, forming an alternate pathway for current and thus risking thermal injury to the bowel wall.

may prevent this type of damage by moving a small point of contact to various areas on the wall. Grasping the plastic catheter near the biopsy port and moving it over excursions of 1 to 2 cm will accomplish the necessary movement.

Bipolar snares will eliminate any wall burn caused by monopolar current returning to the ground plate via the polyp head, but this is never a practical problem during polypectomy. Significant wall damage is more commonly caused by ensnaring and severing an adjacent piece of normal tissue (Fig. 10.18).

Most polyps have a base smaller than the widest diameter of the lesion, and can be easily transected with one application of the wire snare (Fig. 10.19). The maximum-sized base for a single transection is 2.0 to 2.5 cm. Bases of this diameter can usually be ensnared, and tightening of the loop may result in bunching the base from 1.0 to 1.5 cm (Fig. 10.20). If such squeezing cannot be accomplished, the polyp should be removed piecemeal. Because the right colon wall is thin, one should consider piecemeal polypectomy for polyps greater than 1.5 cm in diameter in this location.

PLACEMENT OF THE SNARE AROUND THE POLYP

The endoscopist should obtain a full view of the polyp and its surrounding wall, so that the snare can be fully opened and placed directly over the polyp. In order to accomplish complete loop opening, a tubular view along the colon is recommended, since the snare will only achieve its maximum diameter when the entire loop is fully extended beyond the plastic sheath.

Acute angulation of the colon may make it impossible to fully extend a snare wire, resulting in the absence of loop formation. This can be overcome by using a "mini-snare" with loop dimensions of 3 cm long and 1 cm wide that opens fully in a smaller space. Since the vast majority of polyps are less than 1 cm in diameter, the mini-snare is useful for most standard polypectomies.

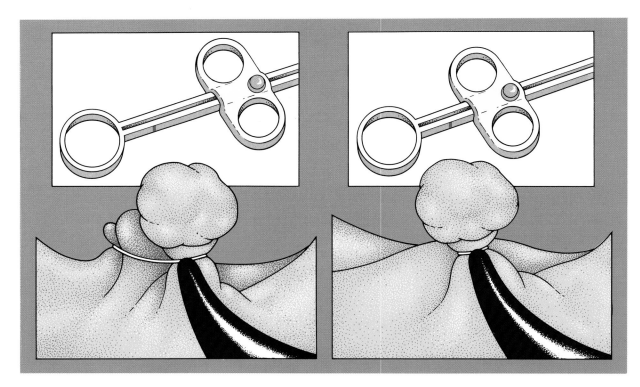

FIGURE 10.18 The snare handles can be marked to serve as an aid in estimating the amount of tissue ensnared. The distance between the handle and sliding bar correponds to the amount of loop extended from the sheath.

Once the polyp is visualized, the sheath is advanced so that the tip is visible; the snare should then be slowly opened. In ideal circumstances, the widest part of the snare loop can be placed directly over the head of the polyp, capturing it completely. Prior to loop closure, the tip of the plastic sheath should be advanced to the point on the polyp where closure is desired. With a pedunculated polyp, the sheath should be advanced to the surface of the pedicle just below the polyp head (Fig. 10.21). For a sessile polyp, the tip of the sheath should be placed at the junction of the polyp and the colon wall.

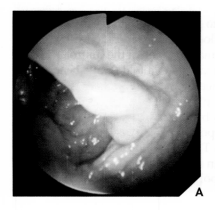 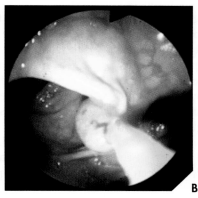 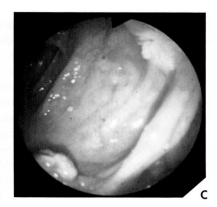

FIGURE 10.19 This sessile polyp is approximately 2 cm in diameter (**A**). A polyp this size can be removed in one resection if its base can be bunched to 1 to 1.5 cm by tightening the snare (**B**). Appearance after resection (**C**).

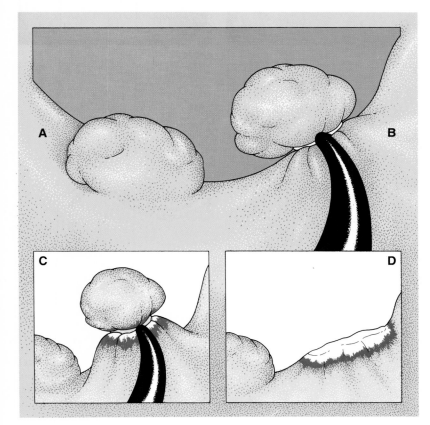

FIGURE 10.20 A wide-based polyp (**A**) can be bunched to acceptable resection size. This bunching maneuver (**B**) often permits single transection of a broad-based polyp that might otherwise need piecemeal resection. Once ensnared the polyp must be lifted away from the wall prior to application of current (**C**). The area of transection will be as large as the original base of the polyp (**D**).

noma. Biopsies of the reddened areas almost always reveal normal mucosal tissue.

GASTRIC POLYPS

Polyps in the stomach may be either adenomatous or hyperplastic (Figs. 10.37, 10.38), and are rarely malignant. Forceps biopsy of the surface of the polyp is often misleading. Small pieces of gastric polyp tissue have a high rate of sampling error. Most gastric polyps are sessile, and may be removed with a technique similar to that used in the colon (Fig. 10.39). The gastric mucosa is more vascular than that of the colon, and slower closure of the snare handle during electro-

cautery ensures hemostasis. Polyps in the antrum and duodenum tend to be rapidly transported from the polypectomy site by peristalsis. To prevent this loss, glucagon, 0.5 mg, should be given intravenously just before resection. This will inhibit peristalsis during polypectomy, enhancing specimen retrieval. With the patient in the standard left lateral position, most resected polyps respond to the pull of gravity, and fall into the pool of gastric juice on the greater curvature aspect of the gastric fundus. Once located, the polyp should be grasped with a wire snare, rather than merely suctioned, to provide additional traction as the polyp and instrument pass through the cricopharynx. During this maneuver, the polyp should be "snugged

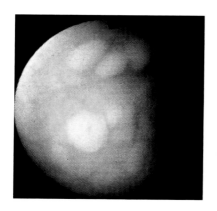

FIGURE 10.37 These small whitish gastric polyps are hyperplastic.

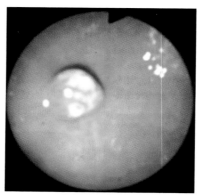

FIGURE 10.38 This small polyp with whitish areas is located on the antrum of the stomach, and was hyperplastic.

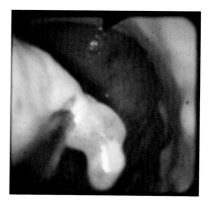

FIGURE 10.39 This multilobulated pedunculated polyp is an adenoma. The wire sheath is in place for resection.

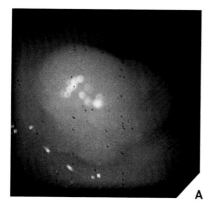

A

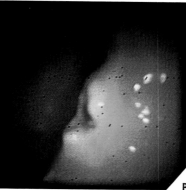

B

C

FIGURE 10.40 A sessile gastric polyp easily resectable with wire snare (**A**). Polypectomy site immediately following procedure (**B**) and forming a typical gastric ulcer 3 weeks after polypectomy (**C**).